30 DAY KETOGENIC MEAL PLAN - INTERMITTENT FASTING EDITION

Intermittent Fasting + The Ketogenic Diet for Rapid and Sustainable Fat Loss

ANDREA J. CLARK

Copyright © 2017 by Andrea J. Clark

All rights reserved. This book or any portion thereof may not be reproduced or used in any manner whatsoever without the express written permission of the publisher except for the use of brief quotations in a book review.

Disclaimer

This publication contains the opinions and ideas of its author. It is intended to provide helpful and informative material on the subjects addressed in the publication. It is sold with the understanding that the author and the publisher are not engaged in rendering medical, health, or any other kind of personal or professional services in the book. The reader should consult his or her medical, health or other competent professional before adopting any of the suggestions in this book.

The author and publisher are not responsible for the results that come from the application of the content within this book. This applies to risk, loss, personal or otherwise. This also applies to both direct and indirect application of the information contained in this publication.

Facebook: https://www.facebook.com/cleaneatingspirit

Instagram: https://www.instagram.com/cleaneatingspirit

INTRODUCTION

Do you want to learn how to lose weight and keep it off? As anyone who has been on a weight loss journey knows, the emotional ups and downs that come with it can be a rollercoaster. We've all tried reducing calories, only to find ourselves gaining weight again and again. Well, I know I have. I know what it feels like to lose weight, only to gain it back again. It's frustrating, humiliating, and discouraging. But it doesn't have to be that way.

I want to share with you the most powerful combination I've discovered for long-term, sustainable weight loss. It's a lifestyle I'm calling Intermittent Fasting Keto diet.

The Magic of the Intermittent Fasting Keto Diet

On their own, both Intermittent Fasting and Ketosis are powerful tools to help you lose weight, boost energy, and feel better in your own skin. Combine the two, and you'll find yourself dropping pounds and gaining a youthful vitality that will shine through your every pore.

There is a lot of magic that happens when we combine these two unbelievably powerful dietary tools.

First, let me talk a bit about Intermittent Fasting. I've been incorporating this incredible tool into my life on and off for the last few years. I've seen some pretty remarkable results. When I am fasting I feel that I am at my most healthy. I feel great, have tons of energy, and my digestion is perfect.

So what is intermittent fasting? Intermittent fasting refers to not eating for a short period of time, between 16 and 24 hours. When we fast for this short amount of time, we dramatically alter the chemistry inside our bodies. It's a simple way to give your body a break from digesting and give it some time to heal.

Normally, when we eat a Standard American Diet (SAD), we are eating high carbohydrate meals three to five times a day. Each time we eat, we have a corresponding spike in insulin. This insulin leads to glycogen storage, which, if we keep overeating, eventually leads to fat storage. In short, the way we eat is making us fat and sick.

But fasting gives our bodies a break. During this break, our insulin levels go down. If we fast for a long enough period of time, we run out of stored glycogen. *Oh no!* If we have no glycogen, we have no source of energy, right? Wrong. Our bodies have a second source of energy that it can use when no glycogen is available.

Ketones are a source of energy derived from fats. When we fast, our liver starts to turn our body fat into ketones. We increase our energy, boost our metabolism, and burn fat. When we fast, our body literally eats its own fat!

Once we eat another carbohydrate rich meal, this process stops, and we return to using glucose for energy.

But what if I told you there was a way you could keep eating filling, delicious meals while staying in this magical "ketone" state. Eating and burning fat? It's possible. And its name is the ketogenic diet.

The ketogenic diet is, simply put, a high-fat low-carb diet. If we eat a high-fat meal, our body stays in ketosis even when we aren't fasting. So, even though we are eating food, we are still burning fat for energy!

If you follow this Intermittent Fasting Keto lifestyle, you get to eat food until you feel full and still burn fat. Does it sound too good to be true? I promise this really works. It is challenging, it isn't always easy, but it absolutely works. You have to make a commitment to yourself, to your body, and to Intermittent Fasting Keto. Commit for 90 days and you will see incredible results. Still don't believe me?

Ok, let's look at it this way. Eating a high-fat diet leads to high levels of satiety. Satiety is just a fancy word for "feeling full". When you eat lots of high-fat foods, you feel full quicker and easier. This, in turn, makes it easier to fast. If you can commit to the lifestyle and avoid all the carbohydrate temptations, this is the dietary change that can help you lose weight and keep it off!

Sound like another fad diet? I know. I thought so too the first time I discovered this. I thought, *how is this different from any other diet*? It might work for six months, but eventually, I will plateau, and then I will regain all the weight. I really didn't want to go down that road again.

How the Intermittent Fasting Keto Diet is Different from Fad Diets

The Intermittent Fasting Keto diet is different from other diets in a few key ways. When you restrict calories for long periods of time, your metabolism plummets. When you try to return to eating 2000 calories a day, you gain back all the weight! Why? Because your metabolism stays low. Your body burns fewer calories after the diet than it did before.

This doesn't happen with Intermittent Fasting Keto. During fasting, our bodies go into overdrive and our metabolism actually goes up. Just imagine you are a prehistoric human. You haven't found food in 12 hours. You are hungry. Will your body shut down? No, because you need the energy to find more food. You will have a boost of adrenaline and energy.

This is exactly what happens when we fast. Our metabolism increases, giving us more energy to get through the fasted period. Eating a ketogenic meal only boosts this process! So, unlike with calorie restricted diets, when we follow the Intermittent Fasting Keto lifestyle, we are able to improve our metabolisms and lose weight at the same time.

I realize that this sounds like a miracle plan. You may be thinking that I have no idea what you've been through. You're hesitant to trust this new promise of a weight loss cure, and that makes perfect sense. Like I said earlier, I've been there. So let me tell you my own journey first.

My weight loss journey

A few years ago, I was 70 pounds overweight. I tried eating a low-calorie diet and exercising more. Eat less, move more. That was how it works, right?

And it did work, at first. I lost 10 then 20 pounds, but I was hungry all the time. I was tired and my brain felt like it was constantly in a fog. My toes were always cold; I'd shiver when no one else was shivering. And I was constantly hungry!

Eventually, I stopped restricting calories. I figured 20 pounds was enough weight loss for now. But what happened? As soon as I returned to eating a normal diet, the weight piled back on! I ended up heavier than I was before I started the diet.

I was devastated and humiliated. I was embarrassed to go out and I didn't want to have my picture taken. It took me a long time to deal with my weight gain. But eventually I learned to accept it, and I knew I needed to get healthy again. But how? I didn't want to restrict my calories only to gain even more weight!

That was when I discovered intermittent fasting for the first time. At that time, I started with 16/8 diet. I started skipping breakfast, and although I didn't immediately lose tons of weight, I felt healthier and happier than I had felt in years. My body felt lighter, and I had more energy for workouts at the gym. It was great.

Next, a friend told me about something called the ketogenic diet - a diet that involves high-fat meals and very few carbs. I was suspicious but willing to give it a try. I made the choice to commit to Keto for 30 days while continuing my intermittent fasting as well.

I won't lie, the first two weeks were really hard. I was always craving sugars, cakes and bread. I felt a little tired and sluggish, and I was always thirsty. When I complained to my friend, he told me just to stick with it, just for 30 days.

After the first two weeks, everything changed. Suddenly I had tons of energy, and my cravings for carbohydrates started to go away. I was hungry less often and more energetic. At the end of those first 30 days, I had lost 15 pounds! I stuck with it for another 3 months to lose all the weight that I wanted to.

Today, I still practice Intermittent Fasting Keto from time to time, not only because I know it is good for my health, but also because I simply love it!

If you're looking to lose weight, boost your metabolism, and feel great in your own skin, then this book is for you. If you've tried the "eat less, move more approach" and just ended up frustrated, this book is for you.

I challenge you to read this book, learn about Intermittent Fasting Keto, what it is, how it works, and how to use it in your life. After you finish this book, I challenge you to commit to Intermittent Fasting Keto for 90 days and see what kind of powerful changes you can bring into your life in only 90 days.

WHY CALORIE REDUCTION METHODS DON'T WORK

It's the age-old weight loss advice: reduce your calories and you'll lose weight. We've all tried it. We start using a calorie counting app. We write down everything we eat. We reduce our calories to 1500 or 1300 calories a day. At first, it works. We lose weight. Some people lose tons of weight.

You add exercise into the mix. Calories in, calories out, as the saying goes. You're only eating 1300 calories a day, and you're hitting the gym at least six times per week. You're a machine, and you're seeing results. Great!

This works, for the first six months. Then something happens. Either you reach your goal, or you hit a plateau. Either way, you finally stop trying to reduce your calories so much. You start to eat a bit more, maybe 2000 calories a day. It is still less than you were eating before the diet, but you hope you'll be able to maintain this new body weight.

You cannot. The weight begins to come back. And despite your best efforts to eat healthily and continue hitting the gym, the weight piles back on. Sometimes, you gain even more weight than you lost!

That is the worst thing about this, the science and nutrition community has known for years that this method doesn't work! The first study showing that calorie reduction doesn't work was released in 1915! Can you imagine? And yet, we are still trying to lose weight by reducing calories.

The Mistake of Calories in Calories out

The hard truth is: calorie reduction doesn't work. It just doesn't. You can try it again and again, but eventually, you'll gain back the weight. But why doesn't it work?

The reason why calorie reduction doesn't work has everything to do with a little misunderstood word: metabolism. People use the world metabolism all the time but they don't fully understand how metabolism really works.

Metabolism refers to the way your body uses energy. Every day, you eat food. Then, your body turns this food into energy. Your body uses this energy for everything. It uses it for thinking, for repairing cells, for building muscle, and for exercise. Metabolism refers to our body's ability to burn calories. If you burn more calories per day, you have a higher metabolism.

And we can do certain things to increase our metabolism and make our body burn more calories. The number one thing that increases our metabolism is eating!

Our metabolism actually goes up when we eat higher calorie meals. So, if you eat a processed sugary food snack filled with empty carbs, your metabolism goes up a little to process that snack. If you eat a nutrient dense, high fat snack, your metabolism goes up even more.

So, what happens when we use calorie restriction to lose weight? It's actually really interesting. When you first drop your calories, for the first weeks, you'll see dramatic weight loss results. That's because your body is still operating at its high-calorie metabolism.

As you continue to restrict calories, you are giving your body less and less fuel. But, your body still needs to do the same things it was doing before! Your heart needs to pump blood, your stomach needs to digest, and your brain needs to think. In order to have enough energy with fewer calories, your body has to start using less energy to live.

When you eat a calorie-restricted diet, your metabolism slows down. This has been proven again and again by scientific studies. When we eat less food, our body slows our metabolism down, and as a result, we feel tired and sluggish.

During calorie restriction, your metabolism shuts down. So, if you were eating only 1300 calories per day, your metabolism tries to slow down to only burn 1300 calories per day. It is trying to match your input!

When you start to eat again, your metabolism does something strange: it stays low! So, even though you are eating 2000 calories again, your body is still only burning 1400 calories. It wants to gain the weight back. Your body will actively try to return to your pre-diet weight.

The Science Behind the Weight Gain

This has been shown in many different studies, most recently in the famous study done on the participants of the hit TV show, The Biggest Loser. Participants' metabolic information was tracked for several years after the end of the show and without fail all of them gained some weight back. All of their metabolisms stayed low.

And perhaps even more devastating, the weight that you gain back will be primarily fat, not muscle. So your metabolism stays low and you are gaining fat even if you eat a reasonable amount of food.

In the end, it doesn't matter how strict you are or for how long you restrict your calories. The simple truth is that calorie restriction just doesn't work. It shuts your metabolism down, for both the short and long term. You will almost always gain the weight back after you stop restricting your calories.

So then, what does this mean? Are we all doomed to lives of obesity and health problems? Should you just give up now before you've even gotten started?

The New Solution

No! There is hope. There are diets and lifestyle changes that you can make that will boost your metabolism while helping you lose weight. It will be a challenge to implement these habits into your daily life, but if you can do it, the benefits will be astounding!

In this book, you will find two powerful tools: Intermittent Fasting and the Ketogenic diet and how to combine them for an even more effective weight loss approach.

Now, let me start by telling you about Intermittent Fasting and the amazing benefits it brings.

QUICK GUIDE TO INTERMITTENT FASTING

INTERMITTENT FASTING AND FAT LOSS

LET'S TALK ABOUT FASTING. IT SOUNDS SCARY, I KNOW. Fasting is intimidating in its simplicity. There are no gimmicks, no rules, nothing fancy you need to buy or prepare. Fasting is one thing only: not eating.

It makes sense that if you don't eat, you'll lose weight. It's obvious. The fact is, not eating for a short period of time can help you lose weight while boosting your metabolism and putting a fire into your days.

How does this work? If you don't eat for days on end, you'll see some detrimental side effects, yet if you fast for 16 to 24 hours a few times a week, you'll see weight loss and huge health benefits. How is fasting different from calorie restriction?

The main root of this is **metabolism** and **insulin**. Fasting affects both of these and in turn, allows you to lose weight in a healthy way.

How Intermittent Fasting Leads to Powerful Weight Loss

First, let's go over what happens inside your body when you eat a meal. You chew the food, send it down to your stomach, and your stomach starts to process it. At the same time, your body releases insulin. Insulin is a helpful chemical. It tells your liver to turn the food into glycogen, a form of sugar that our body can use for energy.

The more we eat, the more insulin we release. The more insulin we release, the more food we turn into glycogen. But what happens to the extra glycogen? If we eat more than we need, we have to store some glycogen for later. Great, the liver does that. It has a limited capacity to store some glycogen, which our bodies can use later when we aren't eating.

Okay, but what if we eat too much, and there is too much glycogen for the body to use? In this case, the liver turns that extra glycogen into fat. As long as we keep eating, we keep replenishing the glycogen stores. If we keep replenishing glycogen, then we never use that stored fat.

In short, when we eat too much, our liver stores extra energy as fat. As we keep eating, we never use that fat, and we just add more fat to the pile. Fat goes in, but we never give our body a chance to burn it off.

Reversing the Fat Storage Process Through Fasting

Fasting is like giving your liver, stomach, and all your internal organs a well-deserved break. When you fast, you allow your insulin levels to go down, you give your digestive tract a break, and your liver does something interesting.

During the first part of a fast, you are still using the stored glycogen in the liver. You are still using sugar and carbs for energy. But, after several hours, the liver runs out of stored glycogen. Now there is no more energy for our body, what will happen?

When we run out of stored glycogen, the liver begins to produce something called Ketones, and our body can use ketones for energy exactly like glycogen! Ketones are made from, you guessed it, fat.

When we enter a fasted state, our body begins to burn our fat stores for energy. Just like that, you've begun the fasting process. It's really quite incredible. You practice fasting, and you lose fat. It's as simple as that.

During this process, two other really important things happen. The first: our levels of insulin go down. Why is this important? High levels of insulin over time lead to more fat storage and increased weight gain. When our insulin levels go down, our body gets a break and we increase our fat burning capacity naturally. According to a 2014 review of the scientific literature, intermittent fasting can cause weight loss of 3-8% over 3-24 weeks.

Next, during a fast, our metabolism gets a boost. In a fasted state, our bodies release adrenaline and this naturally increases our metabolism. The result? You get to burn fat without having the metabolic crash that comes with calorie restriction. That is key for sustainable weight loss.

If you practice intermittent fasting, you will burn more calories, lower your insulin levels, and naturally encourage your body to burn off its fat stores. Sounds like a winning situation. But there are more reasons to include this powerful tool into your everyday routine. The benefits that intermittent fasting can bring to your life are almost immeasurable.

FANTASTIC BENEFITS OF INTERMITTENT FASTING

As we mentioned before, one of the most attractive benefits of intermittent fasting is its ability to promote fat burning in our bodies. If you follow the rules, the fat will melt off.

However, there are many other health and lifestyle benefits to intermittent fasting that might make you even more committed to this new lifestyle choice.

Saves You Money

Most diets include special supplements, organic ingredients, or other expensive equipment that ends up costing you extra money. Intermittent fasting is the exact opposite. There is nothing to buy, nothing to sign up for, and no extra money to spend. If you bring intermittent fasting into your life, you will save money over the long term period.

Saves You Time

We all spend way too much time shopping for food, preparing our meals, and cooking in the kitchen. If you decide to cut out breakfast altogether, think about how much extra time you'll have during your morning routine. Or, if you decide to go for a full day fast, that is one who day you don't need to cook at all! Choosing intermittent fasting really helps you simplify your life.

Cell Repair

When we fast, we give our body a break. Normally, as we follow a traditional eating pattern, we are constantly putting new food and materials into our body. This tells our bodies, on a cellular level, to create more mass. As we eat, our cells reproduce.

But when we give our bodies a break and try intermittent fasting instead, we give our cells a chance to enter something called autophagy. Autophagy is a fancy word meaning repair. During fasting, our cells spend more time repairing rather than building new material. This can, in turn, promote a whole list of health benefits in our body, from weight loss to cancer reduction.

Reduced Risk of Type-2 Diabetes

We've already talked about how intermittent fasting helps reduce the levels of insulin in your body. When you eat constantly, your insulin levels are always high, telling your liver to store extra carbs and sugars as fats in your body. If we consistently overeat, especially if we overeat foods like simple carbohydrates and sugars, our insulin levels stay very high.

Over time, this high level of insulin leads to something called insulin resistance. Basically, we still have insulin in our bloodstream, but our liver and other organs have stopped paying attention to it. This leads to many health problems, one of the most serious being Type 2 Diabetes.

When we practice fasting, we give our bodies a break. During this break from eating, our insulin levels go down, and if we fast for a long enough period of time, we begin burning fat for energy. This leads to fat loss, but it can also help prevent insulin resistance.

By allowing our insulin levels to go down, we stop the process of insulin resistance. This can, in turn, help prevent the onset of Type-2 Diabetes. However, if you are already suffering from Type-2 Diabetes, talk to your doctor before taking on any dietary change.

Heart Health Benefits

Heart and other cardiovascular problems are one of the top killers in the United States these days. And where do these problems begin? They begin with a bad diet. Problems such as high cholesterol, clogged arteries, and high blood pressure can all be linked to following an unhealthy diet.

Intermittent fasting has been shown, in several studies on animals, to counteract some of these cardiovascular problems. This is probably linked to the cell repair mentioned earlier. When we fast, our cells switch from producing to cleaning up. During a fast, our cardiovascular system is given some time to clean itself out and improve things.

Individuals who practice intermittent fasting can expect to see benefits like lowered blood pressure, lower levels of bad LDL cholesterol and lower blood sugar levels. All of these things will help improve your health and longevity in the big picture.

Reduces Inflammation

Inflammation is a pesky little thing in our bodies. It can be a bit confusing because it is both a good and a bad thing to have inflammation. Inflammation is, basically, when your body sends lots of blood and heat to an area to help fight off infection or other issues. It is a tool to help us heal.

In this respect, a low level of inflammation can be a good thing. However, when our bodies are unhealthy, we can develop very high levels of inflammation. If you usually get painful digestion, painful joints, or other unexplainable aches and pains, you may be suffering from inflammation.

This is where intermittent fasting comes into the picture. Again, linked to the process of cell repair, intermittent fasting gives the body a chance to address the various places where inflammation is becoming a problem. When the body doesn't have to focus on digesting tons of food, it can start solving other problems.

Using intermittent fasting to reduce inflammation can help prevent against visible signs of aging and can fight the development of many different diseases.

Cancer Prevention

Cancer is one of the most feared killers in our society today. It is a disease where certain cells in our body mutate and grow at an uncontrollable rate. Scientists are working hard to find a cure for this fearful disease. In the meantime, there are some actionable steps that we can take to fight cancer in our own bodies.

Intermittent fasting's effect on our metabolism can also help fight cancer cells. Certain tests done on animals have shown that intermittent fasting can help prevent cancer by promoting the cleansing and repair of damaged cells.

On top of this, there is some evidence to suggest that fasting can help reduce the side effects of chemotherapy.

Brain Boost

If you take the plunge and decide to practice intermittent fasting, pretty soon you'll start to notice that you feel physically and mentally really amazing. You'll feel lighter and more energetic, and your brain will be sharper and quicker. Personally, I noticed these side effects after just one week of practicing intermittent fasting.

And it turns out, there is science backed evidence as to why this happens! Intermittent fasting and its connection to lower blood sugar and insulin resistance have a whole list of benefits for our brain, as well as our bodies!

First of all, when we are intermittent fasting, this break in the flow of high blood sugar promotes the growth of new nerve cells. This should, in turn, promote better brain function.

On top of that, intermittent fasting might actually help us cope with depression! It sounds too good to be true, but it looks like intermittent fasting increases a chemical in our brain. This chemical helps to fight off depression. So, if you've been feeling lethargic and depressed lately, maybe it's time to start skipping breakfast!

Lastly, on this brain train, intermittent fasting can also help prevent damage from strokes. If that isn't something to celebrate, I'm not sure what is.

The Fight Against Alzheimer's

If you have elderly family members, chances are you've heard of Alzheimer's disease. It's a neurodegenerative disease that happens in the brain, causing memory loss and many more problems. Right now, we have no cure for this disease, so any form of prevention is optimal.

And that is where intermittent fasting comes in. It turns out that Alzheimer's may be somehow connected to high levels of blood sugar in the brain. When we have high levels of blood sugar, this has negative effects on our brain cells, which might lead to Alzheimer's over time.

When we practice intermittent fasting, we allow the levels of blood sugar in our blood stream to drop. This drop in blood sugar has many different health benefits within our bodies, as we've seen, and Alzheimer's prevention is one more. The lowered blood sugar allows our brain cells to repair themselves, giving them the strength to fight off Alzheimer's.

Longevity

Let's talk about something positive. Intermittent fasting might actually extend your lifespan. It's true. Periods of fasting can have such positive impacts on our health and wellbeing all the way down to a cellular level. With intermittent fasting, we might actually be able to extend our lives.

Studies done on rats have shown that the ones that had fasts incorporated into their weekly routines had longer life spans than rats who did not fast.

Since intermittent fasting has tons of benefits for our metabolism, it makes sense that this could promote a younger body, physically and mentally. This youthfulness will, in turn, lead to a longer lifespan. To improve your overall longevity, you should really try implementing intermittent fasting.

But how do you do it? If this all sounds exciting, you are ready to bring intermittent fasting into your life. It is really the easiest trick to begin intermittent fasting. It requires no products, no special diet supplements, and no cost to you at all! And luckily for you, there are several different methods of intermittent fasting for you to experiment with.

DIFFERENT INTERMITTENT FASTING METHODS AND HOW TO USE THEM

Intermittent fasting, as a concept, is really quite simple to understand. You don't eat for a short period of time. After a few weeks, you've lost some weight! Seems easy enough right? But it can be even easier. There are several different methods of intermittent fasting that various fitness gurus have invented over the years. They all have different advantages and one is not better than the others. The key to your success is finding the one that fits with your lifestyle and sticking to it!

I'm going to go over a few of my favorite methods. I want to let you know how I felt while I used them and what the advantages and disadvantages of each are. I can let you know which one is my favorite but in the end, intermittent fasting is a very personal journey. You won't know which style is right for you until you've tried it!

The 16/8 Method

This version of intermittent fasting is by far the most accessible and commonly used form, especially for beginners. When you hear how it works, you'll want to start immediately. It's so simple; it allows you to practice intermittent fasting almost without noticing anything.

And why is that? The 16/8 method is as simple as skipping breakfast. Simply by skipping breakfast and making lunch your first meal of the day, you're already practicing intermittent fasting. It's kind of unbelievable, isn't it?

Let's dig deeper and figure out some of the logistics. This name of this method, 16/8, refers to the lengths of your fasting and feasting windows. Your fasting window refers to the time when you are not eating, and it should be 16 hours long. Your feasting window refers to the time you are eating, which should be about 8 hours.

The simplest way to do this is to skip breakfast. So, let's assume you're reading this book sometime after breakfast. If you wanted to start practicing 16/8 today, you'd continue your day as normal. Eat lunch, snack, and eat dinner before 8 pm. At 8 pm, you have finished eating for the day. Now your first 16 hour fast begins. You go to sleep, wake up tomorrow. Skip breakfast. You first meal of the day happens at noon, 16 hours after you stopped eating at 8 pm. Now, from noon until 8 pm, you can eat as much as you need.

It is really that simple! Try not to overeat during your eating window, and cut yourself off at 8 pm. During the fast, you are allowed to drink water, tea, and coffee, as long as it has no sugar or milk. That's really all there is to it.

The main advantage of this method is its simplicity. It is super easy to incorporate into your daily life. You might feel a little bit hungry mid-morning but for the most part, you almost don't notice you are doing it. I like to drink a cup of black coffee in the mornings. I find that it makes any hunger pangs go away.

The only disadvantage of this style is that the results are not immediately noticeable. You'll feel lighter and healthier pretty quickly. You will adapt to this lifestyle after about a week. However, the weight loss will be slow and gradual. Be patient and commit to trying it for two months.

I'm going to come out and say that the 16/8 method is by far my favorite method for intermittent fasting. It is so easy to incorporate into my daily routine; I hardly notice I'm doing it. I really love it, and even though I'm not trying to lose weight anymore, I definitely still skip breakfast.

The 5/2 Method

Another numbered method! But this one doesn't refer to hours. Instead, it refers to days. This method is another tried and true method that lots of dedicated intermittent fasters really love.

The 5/2 method is also a simple practice and only slightly more difficult to incorporate than the 16/8 method. Using the 5/2 method, you eat normally for five days a week, then include a 24 hour fast on 2 days of the week. The two fasting days can be non-consecutive. So, for example, you could have your fast on a Sunday, and a Wednesday.

For those 24 hour fasts, the rules are a bit different than fasting on the 16/8. During your 16 hour fast in the 16/8 method, you're not allowed to consume any calories. In 5/2, it's a little bit different. During your 2 day fasts, you can eat 500 to 600 calories. For men 600 calories and for women 500 calories are recommended.

So, a typical fasting day might look like a light 150 calorie breakfast, a 200 calorie lunch, and a 150 calorie dinner. Or, you could save all your calories and have a 500 calorie dinner at the end of the day. How you use the calories is up to you, but you should really try to stick to the limit.

The advantage of this method is that you can eat normally for five days of the week. If you are intimidated by the idea of intermittent fasting every single day, this could be a good way to get started and get used to the idea of eating less food.

The disadvantage is that on the fasting days, you might feel pretty hungry. Also, there haven't been any tests done on this method of fasting. That being said, it works for many intermittent fasting enthusiasts.

Alternate Day Fasting

This is the most intense and effective of the fasting lifestyles. It is also the most difficult to stick to. If you have a lot of weight to lose or you're just very dedicated to the intermittent fasting way of living, you can try this alternate day fasting method.

The name makes it obvious. Using alternate day fasting, you eat normally on day one, then fast on day two. Repeat until desired results are achieved.

There are two different ways you can approach the fast days. The first method, you can treat the fasts like the fast days from the 5/2 method and eat 500 to 600 calories each day. Alternatively, you can practice a 24 hour fast on the fast days. A 24 hour fast goes from dinner to dinner. So, if you eat dinner at 7 pm on Tuesday, you don't eat again until 7 pm on Wednesday.

The advantage to this method is that you will lose weight fairly quickly. This is the method that is used in most of the scientific studies done on intermittent fasting. It has proven health benefits for your body, heart, and brain. You'll lose weight, have more energy, and feel great if you can stick to this method.

The disadvantage is its intensity. Especially if you are new to the world of intermittent fasting, the idea and practice of alternate day fasting can be psychologically trying. If you don't feel ready for this method yet, you can set a goal to begin using alternate day fasting after one month or two months of Intermittent Fasting.

Whichever method you choose, intermittent fasting will make you feel better and happier in a surprisingly short amount of time. You need to commit to it, don't cheat, and you will soon be feeling and seeing results.

After just a few days of intermittent fasting, your body will start adapting to the process and will begin to produce ketones during fasts. Remember that ketones are your liver burning your own fat stores? Well, what if I told you there was an even more powerful tool to keep your body burning fat for energy all day long? It's called the Ketogenic Diet. And if you combine the Ketogenic Diet with Intermittent Fasting, you'll be watching the pounds melt away in no time.

QUICK GUIDE TO THE KETOGENIC DIET

THE KETOGENIC DIET: THE WEIGHT-LOSS SECRET WEAPON

The ketogenic diet is the super-secret weapon for weight loss. It isn't easy but it works like a charm. If you fully commit to this diet, I can guarantee you will see the weight fall off.

There are whole communities of people online who are obsessed with this diet, and for good reason. It uses your body's natural functions to lose weight in a safe and natural way. You don't need to buy any special products or take any supplements.

What is the ketogenic diet? Put simply: it's a high-fat, low-carb diet that manipulates your body into burning its own stored fat for energy. How does this work? To understand that, we'll have to dig a little deeper into the science behind our food and our bodies.

The Science Behind Our Food

First, let's talk about the science behind our food. Everything you eat can be divided into three macronutrients: carbohydrates, proteins, and fats. Our bodies need all three of these macronutrients to survive. Carbohydrates give us energy and help all of our organs function, proteins build muscles and cells, and fats give us energy and help us take in vitamins and minerals.

In a standard diet, most of our food comes in the form of carbohydrates. This is especially true of modern diets with their focus on easy grab'n'go fast foods and processed foods. But science has shown us again and again that eating too many carbs is the reason why we put on weight.

How does eating carbs make us fat?

When we eat carbohydrates or protein, this intake of food triggers a release of insulin inside our bodies. As the insulin levels rise, this tells our liver to turn the food into glycogen. Glycogen is a fancy word for the sugars that all of our organs and muscles use for energy. We need this to live.

However, when we overeat or eat constantly, our bodies keep releasing more and more insulin. When this happens, our liver continues to produce glycogen, storing extra for later. When there is no more room for stored glycogen, our liver turns the extra food into fat.

That fat is meant to be stored for later. But later never arrives! We keep eating carbohydrates, we have new sources of glycogen, and we never tap into that stored fat! We just store more and more fat for a later day. But that later day never comes!

If this process is allowed to continue unabated, we can run into some serious health complications. Problems like Type-2 Diabetes come from having too much insulin in the blood stream.

What Happens on a High-Fat Diet?

When we eat a diet that is high in fat, low in carbohydrates, a very interesting thing happens in our body. The ketogenic diet requires you to eat 80% fat, 15% protein, and 5% carbohydrates. This is a radical shift from the Standard American Diet, which is about 80% carbohydrates.

When we stop flooding our system with carbohydrates, our body can no longer make glycogen. At first, our liver continues feeding us the stored glycogen. But this runs out fairly quickly. Then what? Will we starve? Waste away and die?

No. In fact, what happens next would seem to be borderline miraculous if our bodies weren't so cool. When we run out of glucose, our liver begins to produce something called ketones.

Ketones are these nifty things that our muscles, brain, and organs can use exactly like glycogen! Literally, exactly the same way! And what are ketones made from? Fat.

Yep, when we eat a low carb diet, our liver taps into our stored fat and begins to use that for energy! Finally, we are using the stored fat! But if we eat carbs again, we will stop burning ketones and return to glycogen.

That is why the high-fat diet is so important. If we eat only a high-fat diet our bodies will continue to burn ketones instead of glycogen. We will continue to burn our stored fat for energy, instead of sugars. This leads to almost miraculous weight loss.

The most important thing about following a ketogenic diet is really sticking to the ratios of 80% fats, 15% protein, and 5% carbohydrates. The body can turn proteins into glycogen and of course, carbohydrates will knock us out of ketosis. Only if you eat this high-fat diet will you be able to stay in ketosis. If you do commit, the results are truly incredible.

OTHER HEALTH BENEFITS OF THE KETOGENIC DIET

As if the radically fast fat burn wasn't enough of a reason to try a ketogenic diet, there is a whole list of other health benefits that make this diet really attractive. On top of that, they all complement the benefits of intermittent fasting!

Hunger Killer

Because of its focus on high-fat foods, the ketogenic diet does a wonderful job of muting hunger in the body. In fact, when you follow a ketogenic diet, you might find yourself not getting hungry at all during your fasting periods.

During studies, participants who eat low carb, high-fat diets always eat fewer calories than individuals on high-carb diets. So, even without thinking about it, you'll eat fewer calories and lose more weight if you follow a high fat diet. It literally teaches your body to crave fewer calories.

Reduces Abdominal Fat

All body fat is not created equal. In fact, the fat stored in your abdomen, the stuff that gives you a pot belly, is some of the worst for your health. This fat tends to accumulate around your organs and is a solid indicator for other serious health problems.

For example, high levels of abdominal fat can lead to insulin resistance and drive up inflammation. Basically, if you've got high levels of this kind of fat, you're more likely to be sick and tired.

The good news is that high fat; low carb diets are extremely good at reducing this kind of body fat. Over only a small window of time, people who follow the ketogenic diet will see a dramatic reduction in the amount of abdominal fat in their bodies. Sure, it makes you look better. But it is also hugely important for your overall health and longevity.

Increases Good Cholesterol

If you've ever struggled with your cholesterol levels, you'll know that there is a difference between good cholesterol, HDL, and bad cholesterol, LDL. Basically, LDL carries cholesterol from the liver into the bloodstream, where it can clog your arteries and cause problems. HDL carries that same cholesterol away to be excreted.

If you want to increase your levels of HDL cholesterol, the best thing you can do is eat a high-fat diet! Individuals on the ketogenic diet see increases in their HDL and decreases in their LDL. If you struggle with cholesterol, you might want to try a high-fat diet.

Reduces Blood Sugar and Insulin Levels

Remember earlier when we talked about how the ketogenic diet works? It works by lowering your insulin levels and reducing your blood sugar. It replaces these things with ketones, the energy your body derives from fat.

So it makes sense that if you have high blood sugar and are at risk of developing insulin resistance, a diet like the ketogenic diet would be great for you!

Obviously, you should always talk to your doctor first. But there are many signs that a high fat, low carb diet can work wonders for individuals at risk of developing Type 2 Diabetes.

Lower Blood Pressure

Does your doctor give you a hard time about having high blood pressure? If you feel stressed out about your high blood pressure, you might want to consider a ketogenic diet.

It seems unusual that a high-fat diet would reduce blood pressure but it's true! Repeated studies have shown that eating a high fat, low carb diet can help lower your blood pressure, which will, in turn, reduce your risk of heart disease, kidney failure, strokes, and a lot of other diseases and health problems. Why not give it a try?

Brain Boost

The ketogenic diet is even good for your brain! Although some parts of the brain only run on glucose, the liver can create glucose from proteins. But for the rest of the brain, ketones are enough to keep it humming along.

And in fact, the ketogenic diet can be used to treat epilepsy in children. On top of that, the ketogenic diet and its effects on brain disorders like Alzheimer's are also being studied. So, there is a huge potential for the ketogenic diet to have a positive influence on your brain function.

WHAT TO EAT AND WHAT TO AVOID ON A KETO DIET

Now that I've convinced you of the miracle of the ketogenic diet, let's get down to business - what to eat and what not to eat on a ketogenic diet.

The ketogenic diet breaks down like this: your overall calorie consumption each day should be 80% fat, 15% protein, and only 5% net carbohydrates. Net carbohydrates refer to total carbohydrates minus carbohydrates from fiber. Basically, the carbs from fiber don't count so you can subtract them from total carbs to get your net carbs. You want to be eating about 20 net carbs per day.

The best way to understand the dietary requirements of the ketogenic diet are to imagine a ketogenic food pyramid. This is a food pyramid the likes of which you've never seen before. Forget everything you think you know about food pyramids and let's start from the beginning.

If you imagine the ketogenic food pyramid, the base of the pyramid is all your high-fat foods and meats. These ingredients will make up the base of every meal you eat on the ketogenic diet. This includes fatty meats like pork belly, fatty tuna, marbled steaks, and any other fatty cut. It also includes eggs, chicken wings and legs, lard, coconut oil, and even some fatty plant-based foods like avocados and vegetable oils.

When choosing high-fat foods, be wary of meats that have been cured in sweet marinades. A sweet bacon or other cured meat might seem high in fat, but the added sugar could throw off your ratio.

Next up in the pyramid comes your leaner meats and dark, non-starchy vegetables. Lean meats include most seafood and chicken, turkey, and other cuts that have very little fat. Be wary of some shellfish as they have a surprising amount of carbohydrates. You want to include these in your diet but not as often as the fatty meats and other high-fat options.

For vegetables, the best choices are non-starchy, dark, leafy green vegetables. Lettuce, chard, kale, and cauliflower are all solid choices. After those come your nightshades like tomatoes, mushrooms, and eggplants, as well as other veggies. Stay away from potatoes, sweet potatoes, and other high carb plant based foods.

High-fat dairy items like full-fat milk and cheese can be enjoyed on the ketogenic diet but they shouldn't make up the majority of your meals. Yogurt is a disputed territory. Most store brand yogurts contain a lot of extra sugar and ought to be avoided.

At the very top of the pyramid come nuts, seeds, and berries. These have a higher carbohydrate content and should be eaten in moderation. Consider them as your special reward treats on especially high-fat days.

That's basically the skinny on it. Focus on eating high-fat foods, meats, and pairing them with plenty of dark leafy green vegetables. There are many tips and tricks that you can use to get the most out of Keto but in general just following the high-fat diet should be enough to make you love it after just a few weeks.

Get through the first two weeks and you'll quickly start to notice changes in your body composition and weight loss. You'll be hooked by week three, I promise.

The Takeaway: The Combination is Greater than the Sum of its Parts

Both intermittent fasting and the ketogenic diet are powerful tools that will help you lose weight and gain energy quickly and relatively painlessly. Both use your own body's natural processes to eliminate fat storage and boost your metabolism.

In the next chapter, I'm going to talk more specifically about what happens when you combine these two powerful weight loss tools, and what you can expect to experience during the first weeks and months you try Intermittent Fasting Keto!

COMBINIG INTERMITTENT FASTING AND THE KETOGENIC DIET FOR ULTIMATE WEIGHT LOSS

Now that you understand the basics of intermittent fasting and the Ketogenic diet as two separate entities, let's talk about what happens when you combine the two.

If I haven't already made it obvious, these two eating habits are incredibly compatible. When you start to use them together, some really amazing things start to happen. The main reason why it makes sense to combine intermittent fasting with keto is that it is so effortless.

When you eat a high-fat, low-carb diet, you are sending signals to your brain to feel full more quickly. People following a ketogenic diet report naturally eating less because they just aren't hungry.

Now, think about intermittent fasting. What is your biggest fear before you begin fasting? Probably that you will feel hungry. Well, if you're already on a ketogenic diet, you will naturally not feel as hungry thus making the fasting period much easier. People following a Ketogenic diet report that they sometimes find themselves following intermittent fasting protocols unintentionally because they just aren't hungry.

The combination of intermittent fasting with the Ketogenic diet will provide incredible weight loss results in a fairly short time span. Literally, the fat will melt right off of your body. The truly incredible thing is that after you reach your goal weight and you start to eat a more moderate diet again, the weight will not come piling back on. As long as you don't overeat, your weight loss will remain sustainable. So you might ask, *how is this different from a calorie restricted diet?*

When we follow a calorie restricted diet, like one from the "calories in, calories out" model of weight loss, we do more damage than good to our bodies. We restrict our calories down to an incredibly low number, sometimes as low as 1200 calories per day, and expect our bodies to keep performing at their normal metabolic level.

Of course, this doesn't happen. When we restrict our calories that low, our metabolism needs to lower itself as well. Because our bodies cannot burn as much energy when we eat a low-calorie diet! In fact, people who eat slightly more food, but the right kinds of food, will actually lose more weight and keep it off over time than people who restrict their calories.

Why does this happen? Your body is like a well-adapted machine. When you put more food into it, your metabolism rises to meet the level of input. If you eat 2000 calories a day, your body can burn that many calories in a day. If you lower it down to 1200, then your body also needs to lower your metabolism.

The Power of Intermittent Fasting Keto is in the Ketones

When you follow a ketogenic diet, you don't need to dramatically lower your calorie intake. You might lower it a little, especially if you've been overeating, but you don't need to drop down to anything like 1200 calories per day.

Instead, you are changing the composition of the food you are eating. By inputting only high-fat foods and a minimum amount of carbohydrates, you are forcing your body to adapt in a different way. Your body learns to use fats for energy instead of carbohydrates. This is a natural process, and your body is capable of switching from fats to carbohydrates as fuel without causing permanent harm.

So, if you want to lose weight without causing your metabolism to crash, you can choose the high-fat, low-carbohydrate ketogenic diet.

And when intermittent fasting joins with the ketogenic diet, this is where you see the most intense results. Intermittent Fasting actively boosts your metabolism, especially during short fasts. Why is this? It's an evolutionary advantage.

Imagine thousands of years ago, when humans were hunter-gatherers. Back then, we didn't have reliable sources of food. Sometimes, we might not be able to find food for a day or two. What would happen during these periods of fasting? Do our bodies shut down, making us more tired and lethargic?

No. If we cannot find food, we need extra energy so we can move more and find more food. Evolutionarily, our bodies learned to boost our metabolism during the first 24 hours of a fast. This gives us more mental clarity and physical energy which in turn helps us to find more food.

As long as you stick with moderate length fasts of 36 hours

or less, you will find that your metabolism kicks up a notch, instead of lowering. Break your fast with a normal sized meal of high-fat foods, and your keto-adapted body will continue to hum along burning calories and fat at a high level.

People have the power to lose huge amounts of weight if they can practice intermittent fasting and keto as a combined system. It works on a miraculous level to boost your metabolism, boost your calorie burning, and eliminate fat storage from your body. Now that you understand why this is the superior form of weight loss, let's go over some tips and tricks to help you get started.

TIPS FOR GETTING STARTED

START WITH KETO

This one is probably the most important step. Getting started on Keto is not easy and your body will go through a major transition period. During the first two weeks, your body is learning to burn ketones instead of glycogen. As a result, you might feel a bit sluggish or tired. This is referred to as the *Keto Flu*.

The Keto Flu is not inevitable but most people do experience it. Although you will feel crappy at first, you will feel great in the long run. During these first few weeks, when you're feeling the keto flu, this is when you will have the strongest cravings for carbohydrates.

Don't give in to the cravings! Stick it out through the Keto Flu period. After just a few weeks, you'll be keto-adapted and your body will feel great. You'll start to notice the weight loss and you'll have an easier time dealing with cravings.

If the Keto flu is really bothering you, the best thing you can do is drink more electrolytes. Ketogenic warriors love to drink bouillon, or bowls of soup broth, to help them increase their fluids and electrolyte intake. This is important because it helps your body continue to function properly, to flush itself out, and to adapt to ketones faster.

During this Keto Flu period, you really shouldn't try to start intermittent fasting. Wait until your body is fully adapted. Once you get through this Keto-flu period, your body will be "keto-adapted" which means that all your muscles, organs, and brain are using ketones for energy instead of glycogen.

You'll know you have adapted because your hunger levels will go down, and you'll feel full of energy. Once you feel this way, then you can start implementing intermittent fasting.

Stay Hydrated

This connects with both intermittent fasting and the Ketogenic diet. Whether you're on your first few weeks of Keto or you've started intermittent fasting, you need to stay hydrated!

Staying hydrated will help your body function at its best. It can even help keep your metabolism levels high, especially drinking water first thing in the morning. If you're feeling hungry during the first weeks of intermittent fasting, drinking extra water can help offset that hungry feeling.

And in general, staying hydrated is a huge part of health, wellness, and weight loss. The better you are about your hydration, the quicker you'll lose the weight.

Use MCT-Oil

The "MCT" in MCT-Oil stands for medium-chain triglycerides. This oil is a form of saturated fat that can actually help put your body into Ketosis. It can also help with a multitude of other things such as improving your brain function and helping with weight loss.

MTC-Oil can help you get the most out of your Intermittent Fasting Keto diet. These oils are some of the most easily digested of any fats that are available in our diets. Because of this, you get all the health benefits of the oil quicker and more effectively.

Once the oil is digested, it is sent directly to your liver. There, the oil helps to boost your metabolism and increase your output of ketones.

Including this oil in your diet will help get you keto-adapted more quickly, it will help you avoid hunger during fasts, and it will boost your weight loss potential. Although you can buy pure MCT-Oil in special shops, you can also use coconut oil, which is a natural MCT-Oil, as well as butter and full-fat cheeses.

Get Enough Salt

If you're used to following the Standard American Diet, you've probably heard that you need to cut back on your sodium. This is because people who follow a SAD lifestyle are constantly operating with high levels of insulin, which in turn leads the kidneys to store more sodium, causing lots of problems.

But when you're fasting and eating a ketogenic diet, your insulin levels drop way down. When this happens, your kidney stops saving up that extra sodium and your body needs more sodium to function properly.

Easy ways to increase your sodium intake are by drinking bouillon or by sprinkling salt onto your foods. Try to sprinkle salt on your meats or vegetables and if you're feeling sluggish or dehydrated, drink some soup broth!

Exercise

This might seem like a no-brainer for those on a weight loss journey but exercise can have many different benefits while you're on the Intermittent Fasting Keto diet.

First off, exercising in a fasted state can actually help you get more out of your exercise and gain more muscle over time! When you exercise during a fast, your body will burn the extra glycogen in your muscles, leaving them hungry for more. So, during your next meal, all of the carbohydrates and proteins will flood into your muscles helping you improve your performance dramatically.

As for Ketosis, when you exercise, you burn off any extra glycogen or carbohydrates left over in your muscles or liver. After that, your body turns to ketones. So, by exercising, we encourage our bodies to stay in Ketosis and become keto-adapted more quickly.

When you follow the Intermittent Fasting Keto diet, you should also be implementing a regular exercise routine. This can be anything from going for daily walks to intense cardio and strength training. It just depends on what your capabilities and goals are. The most important thing is to find an exercise you love, and stick to it!

Plan Ahead

This is the secret to diet success. If you head out the door in the morning with no meals prepared, chances are you will find yourself hungry without any keto snacks or meals around to fill you up. Don't be that person. Make a daily or weekly plan to help you stick to the diet.

Each Sunday, sit down and make a plan for the week ahead. Go shopping and buy the ingredients that you need. Then prep the meals and snacks. Having Ketogenic meals and snacks easily available will help you get through the day more easily.

Same thing goes for fasting. Plan your fasts and give yourself pep talks before and after. You can do this, you won't die from fasting for 16 hours! Get mentally prepared for a fast beforehand so you can avoid some of the common failings.

Keep It Simple

This is the last tip, and the most important. The best diet is one that you can easily stick to. Make a plan, include meals and snacks, and stick to it! Keep that plan simple, with foods you know how to cook and snacks that are easily available.

There are plenty of websites out there with interesting Keto recipes and adventurous things to cook. Don't try those during the first month. At first, you'll want to stick to things that are easy and straight forward. Roast meats, vegetables cooked in oil or butter, lots of high-fat foods. Just think of all the rich foods you normally avoid! Now you get to eat them. Wrap an avocado in bacon! Just don't try to make Keto desserts during your first month.

Same thing goes for getting started with intermittent fasting: keep it simple! Don't try to force yourself to do 24-hour fasts if you're not ready yet. If 16 hours of fasting seems like too much, start with 12 or 14. Slowly push your first meal of the day back until you reach noon. You don't want to be hurting yourself just for the sake of a diet. This journey should be enjoyable!

Keep it simple, plan ahead, and you're definitely going to find success.

Takeaway: Your Intermittent Fasting Keto Action Plan

Hopefully, at this point, you're convinced to get started on your Intermittent Fasting Keto journey. At the end of this book, you'll find meal suggestions to help you get started. Only you know which foods will work for you and which won't. Find your favorite high-fat foods and start eating!

Step one is to set a goal. How long do you want to follow the Intermittent Fasting Keto lifestyle? Is this a change only for a few months, or do you have longer reaching goals? Do you have a goal weight? Would you like to be able to lift a certain amount? Your goals will dictate your plan, so set some goals for yourself before you get started.

Make yourself a meal plan for the first few weeks. Think through three meals a day and snacks. Pay attention to when you normally get hungry. Are you hungriest when you first wake up or do you get hungry around 2 pm? Be prepared with high-fat meals and snacks. Preparation is the key to success.

Also, make sure to mentally prepare yourself. The first few weeks of the ketogenic diet can be very intense. Make sure you realize you will have cravings, you will feel tired, you might get discouraged. Be ready for this and have defenses! Remember your goals! Determination will get you through the tough times.

Additionally, make a plan for integrating intermittent fasting. After the first two to four weeks of Keto, your body should be ready to start fasting. Choose a method and make a plan to implement it. If you normally wait 12 hours between dinner and breakfast, try waiting for 14 instead. Interested in the 5/2 method? Why not start out with 6/1 for the first week or two? You'll be surprised how quickly intermittent fasting becomes part of your routine.

Still not convinced that this rapid fat loss lifestyle is the one for you? In the next chapter, we will go over some myths about the Intermittent Fasting Keto lifestyle and hopefully convince you once and for all to make the commitment and try Intermittent Fasting Keto.

MYTHS AND MISINFORMATION ABOUT THE INTERMITTENT FASTING KETO

If you're not yet convinced that Intermittent Fasting Keto is the weight loss answer you've been looking for, you may still be influenced by some longstanding beliefs and myths that live in the health and wellness industry. There are many things that we need to first unlearn before we are ready to bring Intermittent Fasting Keto into our lives. Let's walk through a few of those myths and try to understand where they come from and why they are wrong.

The Carbohydrate Myth

The first myth and the hardest to dispel is the idea that we need to eat a high carbohydrate diet in order to operate at full health. In short, we believe we need carbohydrates to be healthy. Is this true? Not necessarily.

For many years, the health and wellness community believed that our muscles, organs, and our brain relied on carbohydrates to function. As we already discussed, when we eat carbs or protein our bodies release insulin and the liver turns the food into glycogen. This glycogen is then used for energy by every part of our body.

However, what happens when we stop putting carbohydrates into our body? Either because we are fasting or because we are eating a ketogenic diet (or both!) something really interesting happens when we let go of our carbohydrate obsession.

Our skeletal muscles are the first ones to switch over to ketones. Once they've used up their stored glycogen, our muscles switch over to ketones and continue to function normally! This lets our brain use the leftover glycogen.

And in a few weeks, once our bodies are keto-adapted, all of our organs can efficiently use ketones for energy. Even our brain can use ketones for over half of its functioning. For the rest of it, the liver can use a few carbs and protein in your diet to take care of the brain's glycogen needs.

In short: our bodies function just fine on a low carbohydrate diet. This is evidenced by cultures around the world, such as the Aleut in Alaska or the Maasai in Africa, who eat high fat low carb diets and have very few health problems.

So, what are you waiting for? Ditch those carbs and make a commitment to the Intermittent Fasting Keto lifestyle!

The Breakfast Lie

The next most common myth that we need to debunk is the idea that breakfast is the most important meal of the day. We've heard it all our lives. We've heard it so much we ardently believe that it is true. But what if we've been misled?

The breakfast lie comes from a simple concept: when we eat food, our body has to boost our metabolism and burn more calories in order to digest the food. This is true. And for a long time, health professionals thought that this meant you need to eat breakfast early to kickstart your metabolism. Or that you should eat six small meals throughout the day to keep your metabolism humming. And while this can work for some people, it isn't exactly the full picture.

The fact is, if you eat 2000 calories, your body will burn 2000 calories, it doesn't matter when you eat it. So, if you eat 500 calories 4 times per day, or you eat 1000 calories twice per day, your body will burn the same amount of calories! It has the same effect on your metabolism.

So, the same goes for breakfast. We believed that we needed to eat food early in order to boost our metabolism. But your metabolism gets that same boost whether your first meal is at 8 am or 12 pm. Why not give intermittent fasting a shot?

When we are eating constantly, our body is constantly in building mode. We are digesting food and turning it into new cells. But when we fast, we let our body change its function. We switch from build mode to autophagy or repair mode. Let your body heal itself, give it a break and try fasting.

The Exercise Myth

The exercise myth refers to the idea that we must eat a high carb meal before we exercise, or else we will be too exhausted and won't make the most out of our workout. I'll be honest, as a weight lifter and exercise enthusiast, this was one of my biggest fears before I began my intermittent fasting journey.

But repeated studies have shown this fear to be unfounded. I was worried that if I exercised while fasting, I would feel tired and my body would burn my muscles for energy.

Surely exercising while fasting would lead to muscle loss, right?

Nope! Instead, exercising in a fasted state has been shown to improve performance and lead to better gains in speed, agility, and strength over time. When you exercise in a fasted state, your muscles burn through their glycogen stores and switch over to ketones. This primes them to receive nutrition after the workout. In fact, it makes your body much more receptive to your post workout meal.

But what about on a ketogenic diet? If the body can turn protein into glycogen, surely our body will eat our own muscles to make up for the lack of carbohydrates during exercise?

Also not true! Since our skeletal muscles are the first to switch over to ketones, our body doesn't consume our own muscles for food. If you think about it from an evolutionary perspective, that would make no sense! Instead, our body is very efficient at switching to ketones when there is no more stored glycogen. Exercise in a fasting state can actually help you become keto-adapted quickly.

Although you may feel slugging and tired during the first few days or weeks of following intermittent fasting and a ketogenic diet, over time your body will adapt and you will see impressive gains in speed, agility, and overall fitness.

The Starvation Mode Myth

The starvation mode myth refers to the idea is that if we don't eat for a short time, our body will hold on to more calories and our metabolisms will lower because there are fewer calories coming in.

Sound familiar? This is actually what happens over time if you follow a calorie restriction diet! When you eat a restricted number of calories for a long time, your body lowers its metabolism to cope with having so little fuel. So, even if you are eating six meals a day, if those meals don't include enough fuel, your body will shut down and stop burning calories.

Why doesn't the same thing happen during intermittent fasting?

During intermittent fasting, we stop consuming calories for a short time. In fact, studies have shown that even after a 48 hour fast, there has been no negative impact on people's cognitive function, sleep, or mood!

During a short fast, our metabolism gets a small increase, giving us more energy to find more food. Only after 84 hours of fasting does our metabolism start to shut down. As long as you end your fast with a hearty and healthy meal, you won't feel any of these negative side effects.

If you follow an Intermittent Fasting Keto diet and eat a normal and healthy amount of calories based primarily in fat, your body won't shut down, you'll have an increased metabolism and a healthy body. Let go of the starvation mode myth and embrace all the health benefits of the Intermittent Fasting Keto lifestyle.

30 DAY INTERMITTENT FASTING KETO MEAL PLAN

Now you have all the knowledge needed for the Intermittent Fasting Keto diet, it's time to kick-start your weight loss with this 30-day Keto meal plan!

This meal plan is meant to guide you through 30-day of eating a ketogenic diet while practicing 16/8 fasting pattern. With this in mind, this plan doesn't include breakfast or mid-morning snack. You can adjust the fasting window to fit your needs, but these meals can fit into any time slot of the day.

Our main goal here is to stay simple as simplicity is key to success. You will thus find only easy recipes with easy-to-find ingredients.

In this section, you will find weekly meal plans with lunch, snack and dinner.

Weekday Breakfast

Since we are practicing the 16/8 Intermittent Fasting, we won't eat anything that includes calories in the morning. However, black coffee or any kind of tea with no sugar is allowed. If you want, you can add stevia or other natural sugar substitute. You may also drink lemon water that contains no sugar.

Weekday Lunch

For lunch, we will keep it simple. Most of the time, it will be salad, meat or something that's easy to be put into a container and bring to work.

Weekday Snack

The key to success in this 30-day keto meal plan is that you don't get hungry. Therefore, I highly suggest that you bring some snacks with you everyday to get you through the cravings. It can be as easy as pork rinds, beef jerky or fat bombs. Just remember to always be prepared so you don't go crazy and end up eating things you're not supposed to eat.

Weekday Dinner

Dinner will be something that is high on the fat and moderate on the protein. Most of them are quick and easy to prepare. Just make sure to cook ahead if it's a slow cooker recipe.

Weekend Meals

After a busy week, it is time to give yourself a treat. You

will see in the meal plan that on the 6th and 7th days (Saturday and Sunday), we usually have something a little special that will satisfy your cravings.

How to Use the 30-day Meal Plan

- Check the weekly meal plan and recipes beforehand and have all your ingredients prepared.
- Customize the meal plan: if there are recipes or certain ingredients you don't like, feel free to replace them by other recipes or ingredients that are keto-friendly.
- For weekday lunches and snacks, make them the night and store them in the containers before so you can just grab them when you go to work. You may also consider one or two meal prepping sections during the week. You can even pack dinner leftovers as lunch the following day.

WEEK ONE MEAL PLAN

DAY 1 (MONDAY)

- Breakfast: Black Coffee or Tea
- Lunch: Avocado Caesar Salad
- Snack: Mixed Roasted Nuts
- Dinner: Cauliflower Mac & Cheese

Day 2 (Tuesday)

- Breakfast: Black Coffee or Tea
- Lunch: Grilled Salmon & Asparagus
- Snack: Pork rinds
- Dinner: Chicken Broccoli Stir-Fry

Day 3 (Wednesday)

- Breakfast: Black Coffee or Tea
- Lunch: Taco salad
- Snack: Parmesan Chips
- Dinner: Dijon Mustard Chicken with vegetables (make more and save some for the lunch next day)

Day 4 (Thursday)

- Breakfast: Black Coffee or Tea
- Lunch: Cauliflower rice + Dijon Mustard Chicken and vegetables (Leftover from the night before)
- Snack: Parmesan Chips
- Dinner: Lettuce Wrap Cheeseburger

Day 5 (Friday)

- Breakfast: Black Coffee or Tea
- Lunch: Thai Zoodles (Pad Thai)
- Snack: Dark chocolate
- Dinner: Spaghetti Squash Burrito Bowls

Day 6 (Saturday)

- Breakfast: Black Coffee or Tea
- Lunch: Sausage Casserole
- Snack: Easy Keto Vanilla Ice Cream
- Dinner: Crockpot Beef Stew

Day 7 (Sunday)

- Breakfast: Black Coffee or Tea
- Lunch: Oven Roasted Brussels Sprouts with Bacon and Cheese
- Snack: Easy Keto Vanilla Ice Cream
- Dinner: Baked Buffalo Chicken Tender

WEEK TWO MEAL PLAN

Day 8 (Monday)

- Breakfast: Black Coffee or Tea
- Lunch: Easy Tuna Salad
- Snack: Kale Chips
- Dinner: Thai Chicken Coconut Soup (Tom Kha Gai)

Day 9 (Tuesday)

- Breakfast: Black Coffee or Tea
- Lunch: Fajitas bowl
- Snack: Pork rinds
- Dinner: Chicken Broccoli Stir-Fry (make more and save some for the lunch next day)

Day 10 (Wednesday)

- Breakfast: Black Coffee or Tea
- Lunch: Cauliflower rice + Chicken Broccoli Stir-Fry (Leftover from the night before)
- Snack: Dark chocolate

- Dinner: Bacon Cheese Burger Soup

Day 11 (Thursday)

- Breakfast: Black Coffee or Tea
- Lunch: Roasted Chicken Thigh & Veggies
- Snack: Kale Chips
- Dinner: Cheesy Zucchini Gratin

Day 12 (Friday)

- Breakfast: Black Coffee or Tea
- Lunch: Cilantro Lime Shrimp Scampi with Zucchini Noodles
- Snack: Mixed berries
- Dinner: Mexican Meatloaf

Day 13 (Saturday)

- Breakfast: Black Coffee or Tea
- Lunch: Keto Fat Head Pizza with Pepperoni
- Snack: Keto Brownies
- Dinner: Crispy Chicken Wings

Day 14 (Sunday)

- Breakfast: Black Coffee or Tea
- Lunch: Sausage Casserole
- Snack: Keto brownies
- Dinner: Thai Lettuce Wrap

WEEK THREE MEAL PLAN

DAY 15 (MONDAY)

- Breakfast: Black Coffee or Tea
- Lunch: Feta and Walnut Salad
- Snack: Nut Butter & Veggie Sticks
- Dinner: Indian-style Chicken with Broccoli

Day 16 (Tuesday)

- Breakfast: Black Coffee or Tea
- Lunch: Low-Carb Bolognese Zoodles
- Snack: Pork rinds
- Dinner: Cauliflower Mac & Cheese

Day 17 (Wednesday)

- Breakfast: Black Coffee or Tea
- Lunch: Salmon Salad
- Snack: Nut Butter & Veggie Sticks
- Dinner: Cheesy Broccoli Soup

Day 18 (Thursday)

- Breakfast: Black Coffee or Tea
- Lunch: Grilled Salmon & Veggies
- Snack: Mixed Roasted Nuts
- Dinner: Creamy Keto Butter Chicken Curry (make more and save some for the lunch next day)

Day 19 (Friday)

- Breakfast: Black Coffee or Tea
- Lunch: Cauliflower rice + Creamy Keto Butter Chicken Curry (Leftover from the night before)
- Snack: Dark chocolate
- Dinner: Lettuce Wrap Cheeseburger

Day 20 (Saturday)

- Breakfast: Black Coffee or Tea
- Lunch: Cauliflower Mac & Cheese
- Snack: Pizza Chips
- Dinner: Crockpot Pulled Pork

Day 21 (Sunday)

- Breakfast: Black Coffee or Tea
- Lunch: Keto Quiche Lorraine
- Snack: Pizza Chips
- Dinner: Chorizo Stuffed Poblano Peppers

WEEK FOUR MEAL PLAN

Day 22 (Monday)

- Breakfast: Black Coffee or Tea
- Lunch: Turkey and Avocado Salad
- Snack: Pecan Peanut Butter Bars
- Dinner: Grilled Tri-Tip Steak

Day 23 (Tuesday)

- Breakfast: Black Coffee or Tea
- Lunch: Cheddar Taco Rolls
- Snack: Mixed berries
- Dinner: Sausage Casserole

Day 24 (Wednesday)

- Breakfast: Black Coffee or Tea
- Lunch: Creamy Avocado Pesto Zoodles with Bacon
- Snack: Pecan Peanut Butter Bars
- Dinner: Zucchini Chicken Enchiladas

Day 25 (Thursday)

- Breakfast: Black Coffee or Tea
- Lunch: Citrus Tilapia
- Snack: Beef Jerky
- Dinner: Spaghetti Squash Burrito Bowls

Day 26 (Friday)

- Breakfast: Black Coffee or Tea
- Lunch: Easy Tuna Salad
- Snack: Mixed Roasted Nuts
- Dinner: Bacon Wrapped Peanut Butter Cheese Burger

Day 27 (Saturday)

- Breakfast: Black Coffee or Tea
- Lunch: Sausage Crust Pizza
- Snack: Peanut Butter Cookies
- Dinner: Coconut Lime Marinated Skirt Steak

Day 28 (Sunday)

- Breakfast: Black Coffee or Tea
- Lunch: Goat Cheese Omelette
- Snack: Peanut Butter Cookies
- Dinner: Garlic Parmesan Salmon

WEEK FIVE MEAL PLAN

Day 29 (Monday)

- Breakfast: Black Coffee or Tea
- Lunch: Fajitas bowl
- Snack: Dark chocolate
- Dinner: Creamy Keto Butter Chicken Curry

Day 30 (Tuesday)

- Breakfast: Black Coffee or Tea
- Lunch: Roasted Chicken Thigh & Veggies
- Snack: Mixed Roasted Nuts
- Dinner: Mexican Meatloaf

AMAZING KETO RECIPES

THE BASICS (5 RECIPES)

CAULIFLOWER RICE

Serves: 4

Prep time: 5 min

Cook time: 8 min

Ingredients:

- 1 large head cauliflower
- 1 tbsp olive oil or butter
- Pinch of salt

Directions:

1. Cut the cauliflower into large pieces: Trim the cauliflower florets, cutting away as much stem as possible.
2. In two or three batches, transfer the cauliflower to a food processor.
3. Pulse until the mixture resembles couscous.
4. Heat a tablespoon of olive oil or butter in a large skillet over medium heat.
5. Add in the cauliflower rice and sprinkle with salt.

6. Cover the skillet and cook for 6 to 8 minutes, until the cauliflower rice is as tender as you like.
7. You can refrigerate the cauliflower rice for up to a week.

Nutrition Facts Per Serving:

- Calories: 42 kcal
- Total Fat: 3.06 g
- Total Carbs: 3.3 g
- Dietary Fiber: 1.3 g
- Net Carbs: 2 g
- Protein: 1.3 g

CAULIFLOWER PIZZA CRUST

When you are trying to eat healthy, you do not have to deny yourself the occasional treat. If you want to eat guilt-free pizza, this recipe offers you an excellent alternative. This cauliflower-based crust lets you enjoy your favorite pizza while letting you stick to your Ketogenic diet lifestyle.

Serves: 1 pizza crust

Prep time: 20 min

Cook time: 30 min

Ingredients:

- 1 piece cauliflower head, stalk removed
- ¼ cup Parmesan, grated
- ½ cup mozzarella, shredded
- ½ tsp kosher salt
- ½ tsp oregano, dried
- ¼ tsp garlic powder
- 2 eggs, beaten lightly

Directions:

1. Preheat oven to 400°F (205°C). Use parchment paper to line a baking sheet.
2. Cut the cauliflower head into florets. In a food processor, pulse the cauliflower until fine.
3. Place the cauliflower in a steamer basket. Steam it and drain well. Allow to cool.
4. In a bowl, mix the fine cauliflower together with the Parmesan, mozzarella, salt, oregano, eggs, and garlic powder.
5. Place the mixture in the center of the lined baking sheet and form into a circle to look like a pizza crust.
6. Bake for about 20 minutes.
7. Add your toppings of choice and bake for another 10 minutes.
8. Serve hot. Enjoy.

Nutrition Facts per Serving:

- Calories: 483 kcal
- Total Carbs: 26.1 g
- Dietary Fiber: 6.6 g
- Net Carbs: 19.5 g
- Total Fat: 21.05 g
- Protein: 49.11 g

KETO COCONUT ROSEMARY BREAD

This coconut rosemary bread is a good accompaniment for paleo pates or soups. The bread's lighter texture, coupled with the aromatic rosemary flavor, is great to enjoy during the summers.

Serves: 10

Prep time: 20 min

Cook time: 45 min

Ingredients:

- 4 eggs
- ¼ cup coconut milk
- ¼ cup olive oil
- 1 tsp sea salt
- 1 tsp baking soda
- 1 tsp rosemary, freshly ground
- ¾ cup coconut flour
- ⅓ cup flaxseed meal

Directions:

1. Preheat the oven to 350°F or 175°C.
2. In a large bowl, use a hand mixer to beat the olive oil, eggs, rosemary, and coconut milk. Mix until smooth.
3. Add the baking soda, sea salt, and flaxseed meal. Mix well.
4. Add the coconut flour. Mix well. The mixture should be dry at this point.
5. Use a spatula to scrape off the dough, and pour it into an oven-proof dish. Use your hands to form the dough into a bread shape. You may also scoop the dough into a baking tin, and use your spatula to spread out the dough.
6. Bake for 45 minutes, or until a toothpick that you inserted comes out clean.
7. Remove from oven. Cool and serve.

Nutrition Facts per Serving:

- Calories: 146.40 kcal
- Total Carbs: 3.02g
- Dietary Fiber: 1.85g
- Net Carbs: 1.17g
- Total Fat: 13.06g
- Protein: 4.87g

KETO SESAME BUNS

While the recipe is easy to make, there are certain variables that can affect the outcome. Use the lightest and finest coconut flour, and use Psyllium powder that's fine, not flaky. It is also important not to use table salt. Instead, use Celtic sea salt or Himalayan salt.

Serves: 12

Prep time: 15 min

Cook time: 50 min

Ingredients:

- 1 cup coconut flour
- ½ cup pumpkin seeds
- 1 cup sesame seeds (Reserve ½ cup sesame seeds for toppings.)
- 1 cup hot water
- ½ cup Psyllium powder
- 1 tbsp sea salt
- 8 egg whites
- 1 tsp aluminum-free baking powder

Directions:

1. Preheat oven to 350°F or 175°C.
2. In a large bowl, combine the dry ingredients. Mix well.
3. Place the eggs whites in a blender and beat until very foamy. Add the whites to the dry ingredients. Use a food processor or a spoon to mix well. The dough should be crumbly.
4. Add 1 cup boiling water and continue to stir until you form a smoother dough. The slightly crumbly dough will keep its shape when formed into a bun.
5. Place ½ cup sesame seeds on a plate. Press the buns into the sesame plate so the seeds stick to the top.
6. On a cookie sheet, place one piece of parchment. Place the sesame buns on the parchment paper.
7. For about 50 minutes, bake the buns at 350°F (175°C).
8. Allow the buns to cool inside the oven to achieve extra-crunchy tops.
9. Remove from oven and serve hot.

Nutrition Facts per Serving:

- Calories: 133 kcal
- Total Carbs: 13.5g
- Dietary Fiber: 9.5g
- Net Carbs: 4g
- Total Fat: 6.5g
- Protein: 6.9g

ZOODLES (ZUCCHINI NOODLES)

Serves: 4

Prep time: 5 min

Cook time: 5 min

Ingredients:

- 4 large zucchini

Directions:

1. Wash the Zucchini thoroughly.
2. Cut the Zucchini noodles using a spiralizer, a mandolin slicer or a vegetable peeler.
3. Set aside on paper towels for 10 minutes.
4. Cook the Zucchini noodles by boiling them, sauté them in oil or simmer them in a sauce

Nutrition Facts Per Serving:

- Calories: 3 kcal
- Total Fat: 0.06g
- Total Carbs: 0.5g
- Dietary Fiber: 0.2g
- Net Carbs: 0.3g
- Protein: 0.43g

LUNCH (20 RECIPES)

AVOCADO CAESAR SALAD

Serves: 2

Prep time: 5 min

Cook time: 10 min

Ingredients:

- 10 oz chicken breast, grilled
- 1 ripe avocado, sliced
- 1 cup bacon
- 4 cups Romaine lettuce
- 1 tbsp grated Parmesan cheese
- 2 tbsp Homemade Caesar dressing

Directions:

For the Caesar Salad dressing:

Blend the following ingredients:

- 1 clove garlic
- 2 tbsp fresh lemon juice
- 1 ½ tsp Dijon mustard

- ½ cup mayonnaise
- Salt and pepper to taste

For the salad:

1. Cook your bacon in a skillet over high heat until crispy.
2. Combine avocado slices, chicken, and bacon.
3. Drizzle with the creamy Caesar dressing.
4. Sprinkle the Parmesan on top and serve straight away.

Nutrition Facts Per Serving:

- Calories: 734 kcal
- Total Fat: 58.6g
- Total Carbs: 17g
- Dietary Fiber: 10.7g
- Net Carbs: 6.3g
- Protein: 41.4g

CILANTRO LIME SHRIMP SCAMPI WITH ZUCCHINI NOODLES

Serves: 4

Prep time: 20 min

Cook time: 10 min

Ingredients:

- 2 tbsp unsalted butter
- 1 lb medium shrimp, shelled and deveined
- 2 cloves garlic, minced
- ½ tsp red pepper flakes
- ¼ cup chicken stock
- Juice of 1 lemon
- 4 medium zucchini, spiralized
- 2 tbsp freshly grated Parmesan
- Chopped parsley, for garnish

Directions:

1. Melt butter in a large skillet over medium heat.
2. Add the garlic and red pepper flakes and cook for 1 minute, stirring constantly.

3. Add shrimp. Cook for about 3 minutes.
4. Stir in chicken stock and lemon juice.
5. Add the zucchini noodles and cook, stirring occasionally, for 2 minutes.
6. Season with salt and pepper
7. Garnish with Parmesan and parsley.
8. Serve immediately.

Nutrition Facts Per Serving:

- Calories: 162 kcal
- Total Fat: 7.45g
- Total Carbs: 5.71g
- Dietary Fiber: 0.8g
- Net Carbs: 4.91g
- Protein: 18.14g

CITRUS TILAPIA

Serves: 4

Prep time: 10 min

Cook time: 30 min

Ingredients:

- 4 tilapia fillets
- 2 garlic cloves, minced
- 2 tbsp butter, melted
- 1 tbsp of lime juice
- Juice of 1 lemon
- Salt and pepper, to taste
- 2 tsp of chopped parsley

Directions:

1. Wash and clean the tilapia.
2. Preheat the oven to 375 °F or 190°C.
3. In a bowl, mix lime juice, lemon juice, butter, garlic, parsley, salt, and pepper.
4. Place the tilapia fillets in a baking dish.

5. Pour the sauce over tilapia.
6. Bake for 30 minutes.
7. Serve with salad or steamed asparagus.

Nutrition Facts Per Serving:

- Calories: 173 kcal
- Total Fat: 7.81g
- Total Carbs: 2.8g
- Dietary Fiber: 0.3g
- Net Carbs: 2.5g
- Protein: 23.69g

CHEDDAR TACO ROLLS

Serves: 4

Prep time: 15 min

Cook time: 30 min

Ingredients:

- 2 ½ cups cheddar cheese
- 1 lb ground beef
- ¼ cup tomatoes, chopped
- ½ of an avocado, chopped
- 2 tsp taco sauce
- ½ tsp onion powder
- ½ tsp garlic salt
- ½ tsp ground cumin
- ¼ tsp cayenne pepper
- 1 can tomato sauce
- chopped cilantro

Directions:

1. Preheat oven to 400°F or 200°C.

2. Heat a large skillet over medium-high heat. Cook beef in the hot skillet until browned, about 5 to 7 minutes.
3. Season beef with onion powder, garlic salt, and cumin.
4. Pour tomato sauce over the beef, stir to coat, and simmer until thickened, about 5 minutes.
5. Cover a medium baking sheet with parchment paper and grease with a cooking spray.
6. Add shredded cheddar cheese to cover the baking sheet.
7. Bake for about 15 minutes, or until the cheese bubbles.
8. Remove from oven.
9. Add seasoned taco meat on top of the cheddar and bake for another 6-8 minutes or until hot.
10. Remove from oven and remove from baking pan by holding the sides of the parchment paper.
11. Top with tomatoes, avocados and chopped cilantro (or other toppings you like).
12. Using a pizza cutter, slice top to bottom and make 4 slices.
13. Roll each slice to form the taco rolls.
14. Serve with a simple salad.

<u>Nutrition Facts Per Serving:</u>

- Calories: 583 kcal
- Total Fat: 40.39g
- Total Carbs: 5.82g
- Dietary Fiber: 2.9g
- Net Carbs: 2.92g
- Protein: 48.28g

CREAMY AVOCADO PESTO ZOODLES WITH BACON

Serves: 4

Prep time: 10 min

Cook time: 15 min

Ingredients:

- 4 large zucchini, spiralized
- 1 tbsp olive oil
- 6 slices of uncooked bacon
- ½ cup grated Parmesan cheese, to garnish

For the Pesto:

- 2 ripe avocados
- 1 cup fresh basil leaves
- 3 cloves garlic
- ¼ cup pine nuts
- 1 tbsp lemon juice
- 1 tsp sea salt
- 2 tbsp olive oil

Directions:

1. Spiralize your zucchini and set aside on paper towels.
2. In a food processor, add avocados, basil leaves, garlic, pine nuts, lemon juice and sea salt. Blend for 20-30 seconds. Next, add olive oil and blend until creamy.
3. Cook bacon in a skillet over medium heat until crisp. Place bacon on a plate lined with paper towels to dry. Wait until the bacon cools and crumble with your hands.
4. Heat 1 tablespoon olive oil to a large skillet over medium high heat. Toss in zucchini noodles and cook for about 2 minutes until tender.
5. Add zucchini noodles to a large mixing bowl and toss with avocado pesto to coat.
6. Serve with bacon crumbles and grated Parmesan cheese.
7. Enjoy!

Nutrition Facts Per Serving:

- Calories: 526 kcal
- Total Fat: 49.52g
- Total Carbs: 13.25g
- Dietary Fiber: 7.3g
- Net Carbs: 5.95g
- Protein: 12.2g

EASY TUNA SALAD

Serves: 2

Prep time: 10 min

Cook time: 0 min

Ingredients:

- 2 (15 oz) can tuna in oil, drained
- 2 large boiled eggs, chopped
- ½ cucumber, sliced
- 1 small/medium red onion, thinly sliced
- ½ small bunch of cilantro, chopped
- 2 tbsp Mayo
- 2 tsp Dijon Mustard
- 2 tbsp lemon juice, freshly squeezed
- 1 tbsp extra virgin olive oil
- 1 tsp salt

Directions:

1. In a small bowl, combine mayo, Dijon mustard, lemon juice, olive oil and salt. Mix well.

2. In a large salad bowl, add all the other ingredients.
3. Add the salad dressing and toss to combine.
4. Serve and enjoy!

Nutrition Facts Per Serving:

- Calories: 465 kcal
- Total Fat: 18.1g
- Total Carbs: 7.35g
- Dietary Fiber: 1.2g
- Net Carbs: 6.15g
- Protein: 68.54g

FAJITAS BOWL

Serves: 4

Prep time: 5 min

Cook time: 20 min

Ingredients:

- 1 lb skinless, boneless chicken breasts, sliced thinly
- 1 red bell pepper, sliced
- 1 yellow pepper, sliced
- 1 medium onion, sliced
- 2 tbsp olive oil
- ¼ cup chicken broth
- Juice of ½ lime
- 2 cup lettuce
- 1 cup cubed avocado
- 1 cup cherry tomatoes
- ½ cup jalapeños
- 8 oz sour cream
- ½ cup cilantro, chopped

Spices for Fajita Mix:

- 1 tsp dried oregano
- ½ tsp chili powder
- ½ tsp salt
- ½ tsp smoked paprika
- ¼ tsp garlic powder
- ¼ tsp ground cumin

Directions:

1. Mix spices in a small bowl.
2. Heat 2 tbsp olive oil in a skillet over medium-high heat.
3. Add chicken and sauté about 5-7 minutes, until golden brown.
4. Add onion, bell peppers and spices, sauté until tender, about 4-5 minutes.
5. Add lime juice and chicken broth, bring to a boil then reduce heat to simmer for about 10 minutes.
6. To serve, place the lettuce in the bottom of serving bowls and top with chicken and peppers, avocado, cherry tomatoes, jalapeños, sour cream and cilantro.
7. Enjoy!

Nutrition Facts Per Serving:

- Calories: 402 kcal
- Total Fat: 22.55g
- Total Carbs: 18.08g
- Dietary Fiber: 4.2g
- Net Carbs: 13.88g
- Protein: 33.1g

FETA AND WALNUT SALAD

Serves: 2

Prep time: 10 min

Cook time: 5 min

Ingredients:

- 2 cups mixed salad greens
- ½ cup walnut pieces
- 3 oz feta cheese
- 2 slices bacon
- 2 tbsp balsamic vinegar
- 1 tsp Dijon mustard
- ¼ tsp ground black pepper
- ¼ cup extra virgin olive oil
- ½ tsp salt
- ½ tsp pepper

Directions:

1. Cook the bacon in a pan for 5 minutes.

2. Crumble and add to salad with greens, cheese and walnuts in a large bowl.
3. Mix balsamic vinegar, mustard, salt and pepper in another bowl. Next, add olive oil, whisking constantly until well blended.
4. Pour the dressing over salad and toss to coat. Serve.

Nutrition Facts Per Serving:

- Calories: 619 kcal
- Total Fat: 59.6g
- Total Carbs: 10.9g
- Dietary fiber: 2.8g
- Net Carbs: 8.1g
- Protein: 13.7g

GOAT CHEESE OMELET

Serves: 4

Prep time: 15 min

Cook time: 15 min

Ingredients:

- 8 large eggs
- 2 tbsp butter
- 2 tsp olive oil
- 1 tsp Dijon mustard
- 6 cups spinach
- 8 oz goat cheese
- 4 tbsp heavy cream
- ¼ cup scallions, chopped
- Ground pepper and salt to taste

Directions:

1. In a pan, heat 2 teaspoon of olive oil.
2. Add the spinach and sauté for one to two minutes. Add the mustard, pepper, and salt.

3. Remove vegetables from the pan. Set aside.
4. Mix 8 large eggs, cream, salt, and pepper in a large bowl.
5. Melt butter in a large pan over medium-low heat.
6. Pour egg mixture into the pan and cook for about one minute. You may need to cook in 2 or more batches.
7. Spoon spinach and crumble goat cheese over the eggs.
8. Cook for another 2-3 minutes.
9. Fold the omelet.
10. Garnish with the scallions.

Nutrition Facts Per Serving:

- Calories: 506 kcal
- Total Fat: 43.01g
- Total Carbs: 6.1g
- Dietary Fiber: 1.4g
- Net Carbs: 4.7g
- Protein: 24.74g

GRILLED SALMON & ASPARAGUS

Serves: 4

Prep time: 10 min

Cook time: 15 min

Ingredients:

- ¼ cup butter, softened
- 2 tbsp dried basil
- 1 lb fresh asparagus
- 4 garlic cloves, peeled and crushed
- ½ tsp black pepper
- 1 tsp garlic salt
- 4 salmon fillets
- ½ tsp fresh lemon juice

Directions:

1. In a small sauce pan, heat butter over medium heat and cook garlic for 2 minutes. Discard garlic.

2. Spoon 2 tbsp butter onto salmon and make sure you spread it around both sides.
3. Place salmon on preheated grill.
4. Cook on medium high heat for 4 minutes.
5. After one side is cooked, place asparagus on grill.
6. Turn salmon and cook another 4 minutes.
7. Add remaining butter, lemon juice, garlic salt and black pepper on the fish.
8. Enjoy!

Nutrition Facts Per Serving:

- Calories: 607 kcal
- Total Fat: 26.62g
- Total Carbs: 5.95g
- Dietary Fiber: 2.6g
- Net Carbs: 3.35g
- Protein: 82.69g

KETO FAT HEAD PIZZA WITH PEPPERONI

Serves: 2

Prep time: 8 min

Cook time: 20 min

Ingredients:

For the Pizza Crust:

- 1 large egg
- 1 ½ cups grated mozzarella cheese (6 oz)
- 2 tbsp full fat cream cheese
- 1 ¼ cup almond flour
- ½ tsp salt

For the Toppings:

- ½ cup sugar-free Marinara sauce (2 oz)
- 1 ½ cup mozzarella cheese
- 2 oz pepperoni

Directions:

Low Carb Pizza Crust:

1. Preheat oven to 425 F/ 220 C.
2. Place the shredded mozzarella and the cream cheese in a microwave safe bowl and microwave on high for 1 minute.
3. Add almond flour and salt. Mix well.
4. In a food processor, blend the cheese mixture with the egg until well combined.
5. Roll out the dough between two sheets of parchment paper or oil your hands and press the dough out into a circle. Make it thinner if you prefer a crispy crust.
6. Transfer the dough to a baking tray and bake at 390°F or 200°C for 12-15 minutes.

Once the crust is baked:

1. Remove the base from the oven and flip it over.
2. Spread the marinara sauce onto the pizza and top with mozzarella cheese.
3. Top with pepperoni slices.
4. Bake on the upper rack until the cheese has melted, about 5 minutes.
5. Slice and serve hot.

Nutrition Facts Per Serving:

- Calories: 442 kcal
- Total Fat: 17.25g
- Total Carbs: 7.87g
- Dietary Fiber: 3.1g
- Net Carbs: 4.77g
- Protein: 63.16g

KETO QUICHE LORRAINE

Serves: 8

Prep time: 15 min

Cook time: 60 min

Ingredients:

For the Pastry:

- ¼ cups almond flour
- ½ tsp salt
- ½ tsp garlic powder
- ¼ cup butter, melted

For the Filling:

- ½ lb bacon, diced and cooked
- ¼ cup onion, chopped
- 6 large eggs
- 1½ cup heavy cream
- 4 oz shredded Swiss cheese (Gruyere)
- ¼ cup water

- ½ tsp salt
- Ground pepper to taste

Directions:

For the low-carb pie crust:

1. Mix almond flour, garlic powder and salt in a medium bowl. Then add ¼ cup melted butter. Stir until the dough is formed.
2. Press the dough firmly with your fingers into a pie plate.
3. Bake in the oven at 325°F or 170°C for 20 minutes. It's done when the edges are golden brown.

For the quiche:

1. Preheat oven to 350°F or 180°C.
2. Beat the eggs along with the cream, water, salt, and pepper.
3. Sauté the onions in a pan for 4 minutes.
4. Add 2 oz shredded cheese into the bottom of the crust. Then, add the bacon and the onions.
5. Pour the egg mixture into the crust and sprinkle remaining cheese over egg mixture.
6. Bake at 350°F for 35 minutes or until lightly browned.
7. Cool before serving.

Nutrition Facts Per Serving:

- Calories: 335 kcal
- Total Fat: 31.5g

- Total Carbs: 5.4g
- Dietary Fiber: 1.3g
- Net Carbs: 4.1g
- Protein: 10.3g

LOW-CARB BOLOGNESE ZOODLES

Serves: 4

Prep time: 15 min

Cook time: 20 min

Ingredients:

- 4 large zucchini, spiralized
- 1 small yellow onion, chopped
- 1 stalk celery, chopped
- 3 cloves garlic, minced
- 1½ lbs ground beef
- 3 tbsp butter
- 2 tbsp tomato paste
- 1 can crushed tomatoes
- 1 tsp Kosher salt
- ¼ tsp pepper
- 1 tsp dried basil
- 1 tsp dried oregano
- ¼ cup water
- ¼ cup grated Parmesan cheese, to garnish

Directions:

1. Spiralize your zucchini first and set aside on paper towels.
2. Heat butter in a large saucepan over medium heat and sauté onion and celery until the onions appear translucent, about 3 minutes.
3. Add in the garlic and cook for another minute or so, until fragrant.
4. Add ground beef and cook until brown.
5. Add tomato paste, crushed tomatoes, basil, oregano, salt, pepper and water. Bring to a boil.
6. Reduce heat and simmer for about 10-12 minutes, until everything is well combined and appears thick.
7. Stir in the zucchini noodles and let cook for 4-5 minutes.
8. Garnish with Parmesan cheese.
9. Serve and enjoy!

Nutrition Facts Per Serving:

- Calories: 565 kcal
- Total Fat: 38.16g
- Total Carbs: 7.56g
- Dietary Fiber: 2g
- Net Carbs: 5.56g
- Protein: 46.46g

ROASTED CHICKEN THIGH & VEGGIES

Serves: 6

Prep time: 15 min

Cook time: 40 min

Ingredients:

- 6 bone-in, skin-on chicken thighs (about 2.25 oz)
- 1 medium red onion, cut into wedges
- 2 small carrots, peeled and chopped
- 4 stalks celery, chopped
- 3 tbsp olive oil
- 3 garlic cloves, minced
- 1 tsp salt
- 1 tsp dried rosemary
- 1 tsp pepper

Directions:

1. Preheat oven to 400°F or 200°C.
2. Pour olive oil into a large bowl. Toss onion, carrot, celery, garlic, salt, rosemary and pepper to coat.

3. Transfer to a baking pan coated with cooking spray.
4. Generously season the chicken thighs with salt and black pepper.
5. Place the chicken atop the oiled vegetables.
6. Roast chicken and vegetables in the preheated oven until the skin is browned and crisp, the vegetables are tender, about 35-40 minutes.
7. Let chicken rest for 5 minutes before serving with vegetables.

Nutrition Facts Per Serving:

- Calories: 407 kcal
- Total Fat: 28.77g
- Total Carbs: 13.27g
- Dietary Fiber: 1.5g
- Net Carbs: 11.77g
- Protein: 23.38g

SALMON SALAD

Serves: 2

Prep time: 15 min

Cook time: 0 min

Ingredients:

- 6 oz mixed leafy greens
- 7 oz smoked salmon
- 1 avocado, diced
- ¼ cup raw walnuts, chopped
- 2 tbsp lemon juice
- 2 tbsp olive oil
- ¼ tsp Himalayan salt
- ½ tsp black pepper

Directions:

1. In a large mixing bowl, add the leafy greens, diced avocado, salt and pepper.
2. Add the olive oil and lemon juice and gently toss.

3. Place into a serving bowl and top with the salmon and walnut.

Nutrition Facts Per Serving:

- Calories: 492 kcal
- Total Fat: 39.32g
- Total Carbs: 15.57g
- Dietary Fiber: 7.6g
- Net Carbs: 7.97g
- Protein: 25.29g

SAUSAGE CASSEROLE

Serves: 4

Prep time: 10 min

Cook time: 35 min

Ingredients:

- ½ lb pork sausage
- ½ cup onion, diced
- 2 medium zucchini, diced
- 3 large eggs
- 2 tsp mayonnaise
- 1 tsp Dijon mustard
- 1 tsp dried ground sage
- 1 cup cheddar cheese, shredded

Directions:

1. Preheat your oven to 375°F or 190°C.
2. Heat a large skillet to medium high. Add sausage and cook for 2 minutes.

3. Add zucchini and onion, and cook for 4-5 minutes or until tender.
4. Spoon the veggies and sausages into your greased casserole dish.
5. Mix eggs, mayonnaise, mustard, sage and ½ cup cheddar cheese in a large mixing bowl.
6. Pour this egg mixture into the casserole dish.
7. Spread the remaining cheese on top and bake in the oven for 25 minutes.

Nutrition Facts Per Serving:

- Calories: 332 kcal
- Total Fat: 26.3g
- Total Carbs: 4.3g
- Dietary Fiber: 0.4g
- Net Carbs: 3.9g
- Protein: 18.9g

SAUSAGE CRUST PIZZA

Serves: 4

Prep time: 10 min

Cook time: 30 min

Ingredients:

- 1 lb sausage
- 2 oz mushrooms, sautéed
- ½ small onion, diced and sautéed
- 1 red bell pepper, diced
- 2 oz ham, sliced
- 3 oz Mozzarella cheese
- 1 tbsp tomato paste
- 1 tsp garlic powder
- 1 tsp onion powder
- 1 tsp Italian seasoning

Directions:

1. Heat oven to 350°F or 177°C.

2. Mash sausage on bottom and up sides of a medium cake pan and bake for 10-15 minutes.
3. Remove from oven and drain any excess grease.
4. Mix tomato paste, garlic powder, onion powder and Italian seasoning and spread onto cooked sausage crust.
5. Lay down onions, ham, red pepper and mushrooms.
6. Sprinkle on mozzarella cheese.
7. Cook until cheese is melted, about 12-15 min.

Nutrition Facts Per Serving:

- Calories: 357 kcal
- Total Fat: 21.21g
- Total Carbs: 16.53g
- Dietary Fiber: 4.4g
- Net Carbs: 12.13g
- Protein: 31.29g

TACO SALAD

Serves: 4

Prep time: 15 min

Cook time: 15 min

Ingredients:

- ½ cup grated cheese
- 2 cups lettuce, chopped
- 1 tomato, chopped
- 1 avocado
- Juice of ½ lime
- 1 tbsp olive oil
- ½ cup sour cream
- 1 tsp salt
- 2 tbsp red onion, thinly sliced
- 1 lb ground beef mince
- ¼ tsp garlic powder
- ¼ tsp dried oregano
- ½ tsp paprika
- 1½ tsp ground cumin
- ½ cup water

Directions:

1. In a medium skillet, brown ground beef over medium heat for 8 to 10 minutes.
2. Add garlic powder, dried oregano, paprika, cumin and ½ cup of water and let it simmer for 3 mins.
3. In a mixing bowl, add lettuce, avocado, and onion.
4. Add olive oil, lime juice, salt and toss.
5. Top with the beef, grated cheese, tomatoes and sour cream.
6. Enjoy!

Nutrition Facts Per Serving:

- Calories: 516 kcal
- Total Fat: 37.47g
- Total Carbs: 9.85g
- Dietary Fiber: 4.4g
- Net Carbs: 5.45g
- Protein: 35.62g

TURKEY AND AVOCADO SALAD

Serves: 4

Prep time: 5 min

Cook time: 0 min

Ingredients:

- 2 lb of grilled turkey breasts, cut into cubes
- 3 pieces of cooked turkey bacon, finely chopped
- 1 cup crumbled feta cheese
- 1 cup cubed avocado
- 7 cups of spinach
- 2 tbsp of olive oil
- 1 tbsp of mustard
- 12 cherry tomatoes, sliced
- Salt and pepper to taste

Directions:

1. In a bowl, combine one tablespoon of water, mustard, and two tablespoons of oil. Season with salt and pepper. Mix well and set aside.

2. In another large bowl, combine the spinach with half of the mustard mixture.
3. Then, add the bacon, turkey, avocado, cheese, sliced tomatoes.
4. Pour the remaining salad dressing and season with pepper and salt.
5. Serve.

Nutrition Facts Per Serving:

- Calories: 559 kcal
- Total Fat: 30.57g
- Total Carbs: 10.2g
- Dietary Fiber: 4.6g
- Net Carbs: 5.6g
- Protein: 60.57g

THAI ZOODLES (PAD THAI)

Serves: 2

Prep time: 15 min

Cook time: 15 min

Ingredients:

For the zucchini noodle:

- 2 large zucchini, made into "noodles" using a spiralizer or vegetable peeler
- 7 oz shrimp (or what ever protein you prefer)
- 2 large eggs
- ½ cup green onion, chopped
- 1½ tbsp coconut oil
- 1 cup Bean Sprouts
- ⅓ cup crushed peanuts
- ¼ cup chopped cilantro
- Few lime wedges for serving

For the dressing:

- 2 tbsp smooth peanut butter

- ¼ cup water
- 3 tbsp soy sauce
- 1 tbsp fish sauce
- 7 drops liquid Stevia
- Juice of 1 lime

Directions:

1. Cut the zucchini into noodles using a vegetable spiralizer or a vegetable peeler.
2. In a small bowl, combine the sauce ingredients and set aside.
3. Heat ½ tablespoon coconut oil in a large skillet on medium heat; make scrambled eggs and then set aside.
4. In the same skillet, add the shrimp and cook until shrimp is tender and cooked through, about 3 minutes. Set aside.
5. Heat 1 tablespoon coconut oil and cook zucchini noodles for 2-3 minutes until the noodles are tender.
6. Add the green onions, scrambled egg, and shrimp back into the same pan.
7. Pour sauce over the noodles, and cook for about 1 more minute, then stir in the bean sprouts.
8. Serve the warm zucchini pad thai noodles with crushed peanuts, cilantro, and lime wedges.

Nutrition Facts Per Serving:

- Calories: 644 kcal
- Total Fat: 39.05g
- Total Carbs: 34.55g
- Dietary Fiber: 5.6g
- Net Carbs: 28.95g
- Protein: 47.01g

DINNER (25 RECIPES)

BACON CHEESEBURGER SOUP

Serves: 4

Prep time: 5 min

Cook time: 35 min

Ingredients:

- 1 lb ground beef
- 4 slices bacon
- 3 tbsp butter
- 4 cups beef broth
- 1 cup shredded cheddar cheese
- ½ cup heavy cream
- 3 oz cream cheese
- ½ tsp garlic powder
- ½ tsp onion powder
- 1 tsp dried parsley
- 1 tsp chili powder
- 2 tsp sea salt
- ½ tsp pepper

Directions:

1. In a large pot, cook bacon for a couple of minutes over medium-high heat until crispy, then remove to paper towels.
2. Add butter, ground beef and spices to the pot and cook for 7-8 minutes, stirring occasionally.
3. Add broth, tomato paste, cream cheese and cheddar cheese to the pot and stir until melted.
4. Cook over low heat for 25 minutes.
5. Season with salt and pepper, and garnish with heavy cream and bacon.

Nutrition Facts Per Serving:

- Calories: 758kcal
- Total Fat: 57g
- Total Carbs: 12g
- Dietary Fiber: 0.4g
- Net Carbs: 11.6g
- Protein: 48.2g

BACON WRAPPED PEANUT BUTTER CHEESE BURGER

Serves: 4

Prep time: 15 min

Cook time: 30 min

Ingredients:

- 1 lb ground beef
- 2 oz cheddar cheese
- 20 bacon slices
- 4 tbsp peanut butter
- 1 tsp garlic powder
- 1 tsp onion powder
- 1 tsp salt
- ½ tsp pepper

Directions:

1. In a large bowl, mix the ground beef and seasonings together.
2. Divide the beef and form them into four patties with your hands.

3. Cook on the grill until done.
4. Add 1 tablespoon peanut butter and sprinkle cheese onto each cooked burger.
5. Wrap up your burger in the bacon. About 5 slices per patty.
6. Place in the oven and cook for about 20 minutes, at 400°F or 200°C until the bacon begins to brown or when it has reached your preferred texture.
7. Serve with lettuce, red onion, or any desired toppings.

Nutrition Facts Per Serving:

- Calories: 850 kcal
- Total Fat: 67.8g
- Total Carbs: 8.13g
- Dietary Fiber: 0.6g
- Net Carbs: 7.53g
- Protein: 49.82g

BAKED BUFFALO CHICKEN TENDER

Serves: 2

Prep time: 15 min

Cook time: 25 min

Ingredients:

- 1 lb chicken breast, cut into ½-inch-thick strips
- 2 tbsp almond flour
- ¼ cup hot sauce
- 2 tbsp butter
- ½ cup blue cheese dip
- 2 large eggs
- 1 tsp garlic powder
- 1 tsp paprika
- 1 tsp chili powder
- 2 tsp salt
- 2 tsp black pepper

Directions:

1. Preheat oven to 400°F or 200°C.
2. Combine garlic powder, paprika, chili powder, salt and black pepper in a medium bowl.
3. Coat the chicken with ¼ of the spice mix.
4. In another bowl, combine almond flour and the rest of the spice mix.
5. Whisk 2 eggs in another bowl.
6. Dip each chicken tender first in the egg mixture. Then, coat each piece in seasoned almond flour. Place the tenders on the prepared baking sheet.
7. Bake the chicken for 25 minutes.
8. Meanwhile, heat butter in a saucepan, add hot sauce and stir until well combined.
9. Drizzle hot sauce mixture over chicken.
10. Serve chicken with your favorite blue cheese dip.

Nutrition Facts Per Serving:

- Calories: 685 kcal
- Total Fat: 43.6g
- Total Carbs: 14.5g
- Dietary Fiber: 1.8g
- Net Carbs: 12.7g
- Protein: 57.7g

CAULIFLOWER MAC & CHEESE

Serves: 4

Prep time: 5 min

Cook time: 25 min

Ingredients:

- 1 large head cauliflower, cut into small florets
- 2 sliced bacon
- 2 tbsp butter
- 2 tsp olive oil
- ½ cup heavy whipping cream
- 4 oz cream cheese, cubed
- 1 and ½ cup shredded cheddar cheese, divided
- 1 tsp Dijon mustard
- ½ tsp garlic powder
- Salt and pepper to taste

Directions:

1. Heat 2 tsp olive oil on a skillet over medium heat and preheat the oven to 425°F or 220°C.
2. Add bacon and cauliflower to the skillet and cook for 5 minutes.
3. Transfer the cauliflower to the baking dish and set aside.
4. For the cheese sauce, combine butter, Dijon mustard, heavy cream and 1 cup cheddar cheese in a medium saucepan. Cook on low heat until everything is melted. Use a whisk to stir in the cream cheese and mix until smooth, and then stir and season with salt, pepper and garlic powder.
5. Pour the cheese sauce over the cauliflower, and stir to combine.
6. Top with the remaining ½ cup cheese and bake until browned, about 15 minutes.
7. Serve.

Nutrition Facts Per Serving:

- Calories: 434 kcal
- Total Fat: 39.11g
- Total Carbs: 6.81g
- Dietary Fiber: 1.6g
- Net Carbs: 5.21g
- Protein: 15.81g

CHEESY ZUCCHINI GRATIN

Serves: 4

Prep time: 15 min

Cook time: 30 min

Ingredients:

- 2 tbsp butter
- 1 small onion, diced
- 2 cloves garlic, minced
- 2 medium zucchini, sliced
- 2 medium yellow squash, sliced
- 1 cup heavy cream
- 1 ½ cups cheese of your choice, shredded
- Salt and pepper to taste

Directions:

1. Preheat the oven to 350°F or 180°C.
2. Melt butter in a skillet and sauté onions until they appear translucent.

3. Add the minced garlic and cook for 1 minute.
4. Pour in the heavy cream and 1 cup of cheese.
5. Simmer until the sauce has thickened.
6. Grease a casserole dish.
7. Place the sliced zucchini and yellow squash in the casserole dish.
8. Gently pour the butter and cream mixture over the vegetables, and sprinkle the remaining ½ cup of cheese over the top.
9. Bake in the oven for about 30 minutes, or until the liquid has thickened and the top is golden brown.
10. Serve warm.

Nutrition Facts Per Serving:

- Calories: 371 kcal
- Total Fat: 33.68g
- Total Carbs: 5.03g
- Dietary Fiber: 0.6g
- Net Carbs: 4.43g
- Protein: 13.3g

CHEESY BROCCOLI SOUP

Serves: 4

Prep time: 10 min

Cook time: 15 min

Ingredients:

- 1 small onion, diced
- 2 cloves garlic, minced
- 4 cups chicken broth
- 1 tbsp cream cheese
- ¼ cup heavy whipping cream
- 3 cups of broccoli (trimmed)
- 1 cup cheddar cheese, shredded
- Salt and pepper, as needed

Directions:

1. In a large pot, melt butter over medium high heat and sauté onion for 3-4 minutes.
2. Add garlic and sauté another 1 minute.
3. Pour the chicken broth and broccoli in the pot.

4. Bring to a boil and then simmer for a few minutes.
5. Use your immersion blender to puree the florets
6. Add the cream and cream cheese into the soup and mix well.
7. Turn off heat and stir in cheddar cheese.
8. Serve.

Nutrition Facts Per Serving:

- Calories: 185 kcal
- Total Fat: 14.1g
- Total Carbs: 5.6g
- Dietary Fiber: 1.3g
- Net Carbs: 4.3g
- Protein: 10.07g

CHICKEN SAUSAGE & VEGETABLE SKILLET

Serves: 4

Prep time: 15 min

Cook time: 15 min

Ingredients:

- 1½ tbsp olive oil
- 12 oz cooked Italian chicken sausage links, cut into small pieces
- 2 cloves garlic, minced
- 1 red onion, sliced
- 1 red bell pepper, chopped
- 1 yellow bell pepper, chopped
- 1 medium zucchini, halved lengthwise and sliced into moons
- 1 cup baby spinach
- 1 cup mushrooms, chopped
- ½ cup vegetable broth
- ½ tsp Italian seasoning
- Sea salt and black pepper, to taste

Directions:

1. Drizzle olive oil in a large skillet over medium heat.
2. Sauté chicken sausage and onion until onion is tender.
3. Add garlic and cook 1 minute.
4. Add zucchini, bell peppers, mushrooms, Italian seasoning, sea salt and pepper and sauté for 2 minutes.
5. Add broth and bring to a boil. Reduce heat and simmer for 10 minutes.
6. Stir in spinach until wilted.
7. Serve.

Nutrition Facts Per Serving:

- Calories: 220 kcal
- Total Fat: 12.49g
- Total Carbs: 12.6g
- Dietary Fiber: 2.1g
- Net Carbs: 10.5g
- Protein: 15.98g

CHICKEN BROCCOLI STIR-FRY

Serves: 1

Prep time: 10 min

Cook time: 10 min

Ingredients:

- 2 cups broccoli florets
- 6 oz chicken breast, cut into 1-inch pieces
- 1 tbsp coconut oil
- 1 tsp freshly grated ginger
- 2 cloves garlic, minced
- ¼ cup chicken broth
- 1 tbsp soy sauce
- Salt to taste

Directions:

1. Heat coconut oil in a non-stick skillet over medium-high heat. Cook chicken, garlic, and ginger for 2 to 3 minutes.

2. Add broccoli to the skillet and cook for approximately 3 minutes.
3. Pour in chicken broth and soy sauce. Continue to sauté for 3 minutes.
4. Add salt to taste and serve.

Nutrition Facts Per Serving:

- Calories: 579 kcal
- Total Fat: 36.8g
- Total Carbs: 9.04g
- Dietary Fiber: 2.7g
- Net Carbs: 6.34g
- Protein: 52.53g

CHORIZO STUFFED POBLANO PEPPERS

Serves: 2

Prep time: 15 min

Cook time: 30 min

Ingredients:

- ½ lb bulk chorizo sausage
- 1 tbsp coconut oil
- 4 Poblano peppers, halved vertically
- 1 clove garlic, minced
- 8 mushrooms, sliced
- ¼ cup cilantro, finely chopped
- ¼ cup shredded Cheddar cheese
- Salt and pepper to taste

Directions:

1. Preheat oven to 375°F or 190°C.
2. Broil poblanos in the oven for about 10 minutes.

3. Cook and stir chorizo in coconut oil for 4-5 minutes until completely browned.
4. Add minced garlic to soften, and then add the sliced mushrooms.
5. Once the mushrooms turn brown, add the chopped cilantro and cook for another 3 minutes.
6. Spoon chorizo mixture into poblanos. Sprinkle cheddar cheese on top.
7. Bake at 375°F or 190°C for 8 minutes.

Nutrition Facts Per Serving:

- Calories: 453kcal
- Total Fat: 30.2g
- Total Carbs: 26.2g
- Dietary Fiber: 5.2g
- Net Carbs: 21g
- Protein: 28g

CREAMY KETO BUTTER CHICKEN CURRY

Serves: 6

Prep time: 20 min

Cook time: 20 min

Ingredients:

- 1.5 lbs chicken breast, cut into large chunks
- 2 tbsp garam masala
- 3 tsp fresh ginger, grated
- 3 cloves garlic, minced
- 4 oz plain yogurt
- 1 tbsp olive oil

For the sauce:

- 2 tbsp ghee
- 1 onion, chopped
- 2 tsp ginger, grated
- 2 tsp garlic, minced
- 1 small can crushed tomatoes
- 2 tbsp tomato paste

- 1 tsp chili powder
- 1 tsp cumin
- ½ cup heavy cream
- ½ tbsp garam masala

To Serve:

- Cilantro, chopped
- Cauliflower rice, cooked

Directions:

1. In a large bowl, place chicken and add 2 tablespoons garam masala, grated ginger, minced garlic and yogurt. Toss to combine and then chill at least 20 minutes.
2. Make the sauce: add the onion, ginger, garlic, tomatoes, tomato paste and spices to a blender, and blend until smooth. Set aside.
3. Heat 1 tablespoon of olive oil in a large skillet over medium high heat.
4. Place the chicken in the skillet and sauté for 4 to 5 minutes until golden brown.
5. Pour in the sauce cook 5 to 6 minutes longer.
6. Stir in the heavy cream and ghee and reduce heat to simmer for 5 more minutes.
7. Serve over cauliflower rice and garnish with chopped cilantro.

Nutrition Facts Per Serving:

- Calories: 319 kcal
- Total Fat: 20.63g
- Total Carbs: 6.25g
- Dietary Fiber: 1.1g
- Net Carbs: 5.15g
- Protein: 26.84g

CRISPY CHICKEN WINGS

Serves: 2

Prep time: 10 min

Cook time: 60 min

Ingredients:

- 2 lbs chicken wings
- 1 ½ tbsp baking powder
- 2 tsp salt

Directions:

1. Pat chicken wings dry with a paper towel and place in a plastic bag. Sprinkle with baking powder and salt, and shake to coat.
2. Bake at 250°F or 130°C for 30 minutes.
3. Next, increase oven temperature to 425°F or 220°C and continue to bake for another 20 to 30 minutes, until crispy.
4. Toss in a sauce of your choice and enjoy.

Nutrition Facts Per Serving:

- Calories: 582 kcal
- Total Fat: 16.1g
- Total Carbs: 5.3g
- Dietary Fiber: 0.2g
- Net Carbs: 5.1g
- Protein: 99g

COCONUT LIME MARINATED SKIRT STEAK

Serves: 3

Prep time: 40 min

Cook time: 8 min

Ingredients:

- 2 lbs skirt steak (grass fed)
- ½ cup virgin coconut oil
- 2 tbsp fresh lime juice
- 1 tbsp garlic, minced
- 1 tbsp ginger, grated
- 1 tsp Himalayan salt

Directions:

1. Take a small bowl and add melted coconut oil, lime juice, garlic, ginger and Himalayan salt. Stir until well combined.
2. Place skirt steak in a resealable bag and pour

marinade over the steak. Let the steak marinate for about 30 minutes. Do not skip this step.
3. Cook the steak in a skillet over medium-high heat for about 4 minutes per side.
4. Serve.

Nutrition Facts Per Serving:

- Calories: 787 kcal
- Total Fat: 48.1g
- Total Carbs: 2.1g
- Dietary Fiber: 0.1g
- Net Carbs: 2g
- Protein: 89g

CROCKPOT BEEF STEW

Serves: 4

Prep time: 10 min

Cook time: 6.5 hour

Ingredients:

- 2 lbs beef stew meat, cut into 1-inch cubes
- ½ Yellow onion, chopped
- 2 cloves garlic, minced
- 3 tomatoes, diced
- 1 cup beef broth
- 2 tsp hot sauce
- 1 tbsp Worcestershire sauce
- 1 tbsp dried thyme
- ¼ cup almond flour
- Kosher salt and black pepper to taste

Directions:

1. Set your crockpot to high.

2. Coat the meat with salt, pepper and almond flour. Place it in your crockpot.
3. Add the remaining ingredients.
4. Cook on high for 30 minutes and then on low for 6 hours.
5. Add salt and pepper to taste.

Nutrition Facts Per Serving:

- Calories: 706 kcal
- Total Fat: 57.8g
- Total Carbs: 8.4g
- Dietary Fiber: 2.3g
- Net Carbs: 6.1g
- Protein: 37.2g

CROCKPOT PULLED PORK

Serves: 8

Prep time: 20 min

Cook time: 10 hrs

Ingredients:

- 1 chopped white onion
- 3 lb boneless pork shoulder
- 3 bay leaves
- 3 tsp pink Himalayan salt
- 1 tsp smoked paprika
- 2 tsp garlic powder

Directions:

1. Turn on the slow cooker to low.
2. Mix together the garlic powder, paprika and some salt in your bowl.
3. Make cuts in the surface of the pork with your kitchen knife and rub in spices.

4. Place the pork along with the onion in the warm slow cooker.
5. Toss in the bay leaves.
6. Cover and adjust the temperature setting to low.
7. Allow to cook for 10 hours.
8. Shred the pork and serve hot!

<u>Nutrition Facts Per Serving:</u>

- Calories: 464 kcal
- Carbohydrates: 2.2g
- Dietary Fiber: 0.6g
- Protein: 43g
- Fat: 30.2g
- Saturated Fat: 11.2g

DIJON MUSTARD CHICKEN WITH VEGETABLES

Serves: 4

Prep time: 15 min

Cook time: 30 min

Ingredients:

- 4 bone-in skin-on chicken thighs
- 3 tsp kosher salt, divided
- 4 tbsp olive oil, divided
- 3 tbsp Dijon mustard, divided
- 1 clove garlic, minced
- 1 tbsp fresh thyme leaves
- 3 medium yellow onion, sliced
- 4 medium carrots, peeled and cut into 4-inch pieces
- 2 cups broccoli florets
- 2 cups cauliflower florets
- 1 juice of lemon

Directions:

1. Preheat oven to 425°F or 220°F.
2. In a small bowl, mix 2 tablespoons oil, 2 tablespoons mustard, 1 tablespoon garlic, and 2 teaspoons salt. Brush the mixture onto chicken.
3. Place chicken thighs skin side up on a baking sheet. Bake for 10 minutes.
4. Meanwhile, in a large bowl, add garlic, thyme, 2 tablespoons olive oil, 1 tablespoon mustard, lemon juice, and 1 teaspoon salt. Add onions, carrots, broccoli, and cauliflower. Toss to coat.
5. Place the vegetables in the pan.
6. Continue to bake until vegetables are tender, about 25 minutes.
7. Garnish with thyme, if desired.
8. Serve.

Nutrition Facts Per Serving:

- Calories: 603 kcal
- Total Fat: 46.39g
- Total Carbs: 12.09g
- Dietary Fiber: 4g
- Net Carbs: 8.09g
- Protein: 34.75g

GARLIC PARMESAN SALMON

Serves: 2

Prep time: 5 min

Cook time: 30 min

Ingredients:

- 2 salmon fillets, around 9 oz
- 2 tbsp butter
- 3 cloves garlic, minced
- ½ cup Parmesan cheese, grated
- ¼ cup heavy cream
- A bunch of fresh parsley, chopped
- Salt and pepper to taste

Directions:

1. Preheat oven to 350°F or 180°C.
2. Line a baking pan with parchment paper.
3. Place salmon in the pan and season with sea salt and pepper. Set aside.

4. Heat butter in a skillet over medium heat. Sauté garlic until softened.
5. Reduce the heat to low. Add heavy cream and Parmesan and stir until melted.
6. Pour mixture over your salmon fillet.
7. Bake for about 15-20 minutes. Add salt to taste.
8. Top with chopped parsley and serve with a simple salad.

Nutrition Facts Per Serving:

- Calories: 480 kcal
- Total Fat: 33.5g
- Total Carbs: 9.4g
- Dietary Fiber: 1.4g
- Net Carbs: 8g
- Protein: 35.5g

GRILLED TRI-TIP STEAK

Serves: 4

Prep time: 2 hrs (marinating)

Cook time: 10 min

Ingredients:

- 1 tri-tip steak, about 2 pounds
- 3 tbsp olive oil
- 1 clove garlic, minced
- 1 tsp ground black pepper
- ½ tbsp sea salt

Directions:

1. In a large bowl, combine minced garlic, olive oil, salt and black pepper.
2. Place the beef tri-tip in the marinade. Marinate in the refrigerator for at least 1-2 hours.
3. Heat a skillet over medium-high heat. Cook 5 minutes on each side.

4. Cut your steak into slices and serve with a simple salad.

Nutrition Facts Per Serving:

- Calories: 693 kcal
- Total Fat: 44.6g
- Total Carbs: 0.7g
- Dietary Fiber: 0.2g
- Net Carbs: 0.5g
- Protein: 68g

INDIAN-STYLE CHICKEN WITH BROCCOLI

Serves: 4

Prep time: 130 min (2 hours marinating)

Cook time: 20 min

Ingredients:

- 4 chicken breasts, skinless and boneless
- 3 cloves garlic, minced
- ½ tsp of ground turmeric
- ½ tsp of cayenne pepper
- 1 tsp of cumin
- 1 tbsp of olive oil
- 1 tbsp ginger, grated
- 1 onion, chopped
- 1 cup of full fat Greek yogurt
- 4 cups of broccoli, steamed
- Salt and pepper, to taste

Directions:

1. Place the chicken, yogurt, onion, ginger, olive oil,

cayenne pepper, turmeric, salt and pepper in a zip-lock bag.
2. Place in the refrigerator and marinate for two hours.
3. Preheat the oven to 350°F or 180°C.
4. Remove the marinated chicken from the zip-lock bag.
5. Spray some oil on a baking pan.
6. Place the chicken in the pan and bake for 10 minutes.
7. Remove the chicken from the oven and turn to the other side.
8. Bake for another 10 minutes.
9. Slice the chicken into small bite pieces.
10. Serve with steamed broccoli.

Nutrition Facts Per Serving:

- Calories: 563 kcal
- Total Fat: 30.65g
- Total Carbs: 6.28g
- Dietary Fiber: 2g
- Net Carbs: 4.28g
- Protein: 63.03g

LETTUCE WRAP CHEESEBURGER

Serves: 1

Prep time: 5 min

Cook time: 10 min

Ingredients:

- 5 oz ground beef
- 1 slice American cheese
- Fresh Lettuce leaves
- 2 or 3 rings, red onion
- ½ tsp Kosher salt
- ¼ tsp pepper
- 1 tsp dried oregano
- 1 tsp Mayonnaise

Directions:

1. Season your beef with Kosher salt, pepper, and oregano.

2. Place the beef on the grill and cook about 4-5 minutes on each side.
3. Once the burger is done, remove it from the grill.
4. Place a slice of cheese on your cooked burger and place it on a large piece of lettuce.
5. Top with mayonnaise, red onion rings and wrap the lettuce up over the top and serve.

Nutrition Facts Per Serving:

- Calories: 601kcal
- Total Fat: 51.5g
- Total Carbs: 6.7g
- Dietary Fiber: 1.2g
- Net Carbs: 5.5g
- Protein: 26.7g

MEXICAN MEATLOAF

Serves: 8

Prep time: 15 min

Cook time: 70 min

Ingredients:

For the meatloaf:

- 2 lbs ground beef
- 2 eggs
- ½ cup salsa
- 2 tsp chili powder
- 2 tsp cumin
- ½ tsp pepper
- 1 cup pork rind, processed into a fine crumb
- 1 cup grated cheddar cheese
- 1 small onion, chopped in small pieces

Topping ideas (optional):

- Salsa
- Shredded cheese

- Sour cream
- Guacamole
- Shredded lettuce

Directions:

1. Preheat oven to 350°F or 180°C.
2. In a large bowl, mix ground beef, pork rinds, eggs, chili powder, cumin, pepper and onion together.
3. Press half of the mixture in a bread pan.
4. Sprinkle with ½ cup of the cheese.
5. Press remaining meat mixture over cheese.
6. Bake for approximately 60 to 70 minutes.
7. Add the remaining ½ cup of the cheese.
8. Cook for another 10 minutes or until cheese is bubbly.
9. Remove from oven. Let cool 10 minutes and serve warm.

Nutrition Facts Per Serving:

- Calories: 372 kcal
- Total Fat: 20.94g
- Total Carbs: 3.26g
- Dietary Fiber: 0.8g
- Net Carbs: 2.46g
- Protein: 40.69g

OVEN ROASTED BRUSSELS SPROUTS WITH BACON AND CHEESE

Serves: 6

Prep time: 20 min

Cook time: 25 min

Ingredients:

- 3 tbsp butter
- 2 cloves garlic, minced
- 1 ½ pounds Brussels sprouts
- Kosher salt and freshly ground black pepper
- 3/4 cup heavy whipping cream
- ½ cup shredded Gruyere cheese
- 6 bacon slices, crumbled

Directions:

1. Preheat oven to 375°F or 190°C.
2. Clean and trim Brussels sprouts.
3. Melt butter in a large oven safe pan over medium heat.

4. Add garlic and Brussels sprouts, season with salt and black pepper. Sauté for 5 to 6 minutes.
5. Remove the pan from heat, and add heavy whipping cream.
6. Add crumbled bacon.
7. Top with shredded Gruyere cheese and bake about 10 minutes, until cheese is bubbly.

<u>Nutrition Facts Per Serving:</u>

- Calories: 304 kcal
- Total Fat: 25.42g
- Total Carbs: 11.16g
- Dietary Fiber: 4.3g
- Net Carbs: 6.86g
- Protein: 10.8g

SPAGHETTI SQUASH BURRITO BOWLS

Serves: 4

Prep time: 20 min

Cook time: 50 min

Ingredients:

- 2 medium spaghetti squash, halved and seeds removed
- 1 lb minced ground beef
- 2 tbsp olive oil
- 1 red onion, sliced
- 1 clove garlic, minced
- 1 red bell pepper, sliced
- 2 jalapenos, cored and sliced
- 1 cup shredded cheddar
- 1 tsp cumin
- 1 tsp chili powder
- 1 small jar of salsa
- 6 green onions, chopped
- ½ cup fresh cilantro, finely chopped
- Salt & pepper to taste

Directions:

1. Preheat the oven to 400°F or 200°C and line a baking sheet with parchment paper.
2. On the baking sheet, drizzle the halved spaghetti squash with olive oil and season with freshly ground black pepper and salt.
3. Place each half face down on the baking sheet.
4. Roast in the oven for 30-45 minutes, until the squash is easily pierced through with a fork.
5. Meanwhile, warm oil in a large pan over medium heat.
6. Sauté the red onion for a few minutes until tender.
7. Add the beef, garlic, cumin and chili powder and cook for another 3-5 minutes.
8. Add the bell peppers and jalapeño, and cook until desired softness. Season with salt and pepper.
9. Remove squash from oven and let cool for 10 minutes.
10. Use a fork to separate and fluff up the flesh of the spaghetti squash and scrape about ½ of the inside out onto a dish.
11. Add the filling to each "bowl" and top with chopped green onions, salsa and shredded cheese.
12. Broil in the oven for 5 minutes, or until cheese is bubble and golden brown.
13. Garnish the bowls with chopped cilantro. Serve.

Nutrition Facts Per Serving:

- Calories: 528 kcal
- Total Fat: 31.75g
- Total Carbs: 20.28g
- Dietary Fiber: 6.2g

- Net Carbs: 14.08g
- Protein: 42.48g

THAI CHICKEN COCONUT SOUP (TOM KHA GAI)

The ingredients you'll need can be found online or in most Asian supermarkets throughout the US and Europe.

Serves: 4

Prep time: 10 min

Cook time: 10 min

Ingredients:

- 1 can (14 oz.) coconut milk
- 1 can (14 oz.) reduced-sodium chicken broth
- 1 lb chicken thighs, cut into chunks
- 1 thumb chunk of galangal
- 2 stalks fresh lemongrass, use only the white part, cut in pieces and crushed
- 6 kaffir lime leaves
- 1 cup sliced mushrooms
- 2 tomatoes, cut into cubes
- 2 tbsp fresh lime juice
- 1 tbsp Thai fish sauce
- 1 tsp Thai chili paste

- Small bunch of cilantro

Directions:

1. Turn on your stove to medium high heat, add coconut milk, broth, Thai chili paste, sliced galangal and lemongrass. Bring to a boil.
2. Add chicken and cook for 2 minutes, and then turn down the heat to a medium low
3. Add mushrooms, tomatoes and continue to cook for 3-5 minutes.
4. Stir in Thai fish sauce and lime juice.
5. Break the kaffir lime leaves and toss directly into the soup.
6. Discard lemongrass and galangal, and top with cilantro before serving.

Nutrition Facts Per Serving:

- Calories: 324 kcal
- Total Fat: 19.73g
- Total Carbs: 16.15g
- Dietary Fiber: 2.2g
- Net Carbs: 13.95g
- Protein: 23.2g

THAI LETTUCE WRAP

Serves: 4

Prep time: 15 min

Cook time: 10 min

Ingredients:

- 1 large head iceberg or butter lettuce
- 1 tbsp olive oil
- 1 lb chicken breasts, chopped into very small pieces
- 3 cloves garlic, minced
- 1 large red onion, chopped
- 3 green onions, chopped
- ¼ cup cilantro, chopped
- ¼ cup peanuts, chopped
- Salt and pepper to taste

For the sauce:

- ¼ cup chili sauce
- 1 tbsp smooth peanut butter
- ¼ tsp ground ginger

- 1 tbsp reduced sodium soy sauce
- 2 tsp fish sauce
- Juice of ½ lime

Directions:

1. Heat oil in a large skillet over medium heat.
2. Add the onion and cook, stirring frequently, until soft, about 4 minutes.
3. Add the garlic and cook 1 minute more.
4. Add the chicken and turn the heat up to medium high.
5. Cook about 3 minutes until partially cooked through.
6. In a small bowl, combine the sauce ingredients and stir until smooth.
7. Add the sauce to the skillet and continue cooking, until the chicken is cooked through, 5 minutes more.
8. Stir in the green onions, cilantro and peanuts. Toss everything until combined.
9. Taste and adjust seasoning if necessary.
10. Spoon mixture into lettuce cups and serve.

Nutrition Facts Per Serving:

- Calories: 426 kcal
- Total Fat: 22.08g
- Total Carbs: 26.45g
- Dietary Fiber: 6.3g
- Net Carbs: 20.15g
- Protein: 32.5g

ZUCCHINI CHICKEN ENCHILADAS

Serves: 4

Prep time: 20 min

Cook time: 30 min

Ingredients:

- 1 lb chicken, boiled and shredded
- 1 medium onion, cubed
- 4 large zucchinis, cut into long flat sheets using a mandoline or vegetable peeler
- 1 tbsp butter
- 2 tsp chili powder
- 2 tsp ground cumin
- 1 cup shredded jack cheese
- 1 cup shredded cheddar cheese

For the keto Enchilada Sauce:

- 1 can tomato paste
- ¼ cup olive oil

- ½ cup water
- ½ tsp hot sauce
- 1 tsp Italian spices
- 1 tsp onion powder
- 1 tsp garlic powder
- 1 tsp ground pepper

Optional toppings:

- Sour cream
- Guacamole
- Chopped tomatoes
- Jalapeno
- Chopped cilantro
- Green onions

Directions:

1. Preheat oven to 350°F or 180°C.
2. Make the sauce by mixing the sauce ingredients in a medium bowl.
3. Melt the butter in a large skillet. Sauté the chopped onion until soft, around 3-4 minutes.
4. Add the shredded chicken, chili powder, cumin and 1 cup of keto enchilada sauce to make the chicken mixture. Set aside.
5. Lay out 4 slices of zucchini, slightly overlapping.
6. Place a spoonful of chicken mixture on top.
7. Roll up and transfer to a baking dish.
8. Repeat the previous 3 steps with remaining zucchini and chicken mixture.
9. Next, top with keto Enchilada sauce and sprinkle both cheese on the entire dish.
10. Bake in the oven at 350 degrees for 20-25 minutes

until the cheese is melted and bubbly, and the zucchini is cooked.
11. Serve with desired toppings.

Nutrition Facts Per Serving:

- Calories: 297 kcal
- Total Fat: 16.45g
- Total Carbs: 4.43g
- Dietary Fiber: 1.2g
- Net Carbs: 3.23g
- Protein: 32.27g

SNACKS AND DESSERTS (10 RECIPES)

CINNAMON CHIA PUDDING

Serves: 1

Prep time: 3 hrs

Cook time: 0 min

Ingredients:

- 1 tbsp chia seeds
- 1 cup unsweetened almond milk
- ½ tsp ground cinnamon
- 1 tbsp peanut butter
- 8 drops stevia

Directions:

1. Add almond milk, peanut butter, cinnamon and stevia to your blender.
2. Blend until smooth.
3. Add chia seeds to the mixture and stir.
4. Refrigerate for about 3 hours.
5. Enjoy!

Nutrition Facts Per Serving:

- Calories: 384 kcal
- Total Fat: 24.7g
- Total Carbs: 28.17g
- Dietary Fiber: 11.5g
- Net Carbs: 16.7g
- Protein: 16.28g

EASY KETO VANILLA ICE CREAM

If you don't have cream of tartar, you can use a ¼ teaspoon of apple cider vinegar, and you can easily turn this dairy free by using coconut milk which will work just as well for this sweet and simple recipe.

Serves: 1

Prep time: 10 min

Total time: 30 min

Ingredients:

- 4 large eggs
- ¼ tsp cream of tartar
- ½ cup erythritol
- 1 ¼ cup heavy whipping cream
- 1 tbsp vanilla extract

Directions:

1. Start by separating your egg yolks from your egg

whites, and whisk the egg whites with the cream of tartar. The egg whites will begin to thicken, and as they do you're going to need to add the Erythritol. They should start to form stiff peaks, and you'll need to keep whisking until they do.
2. Take another bowl, and start to whisk your cream. Soft peaks should start to form as the whisk is removed, but you'll need to be careful not to over whisk the cream.
3. In a third bowl, combine your egg yolks with the vanilla.
4. Now you can fold the whisked egg whites into the now whipped cream.
5. Add in your egg yolk mixture, and continue to gently fold with a spatula until thoroughly combined.
6. Place it in a pan, preferably a loaf pan, and let it sit. All hands on time is done, but it'll need to sit for about two hours.

Nutrition Facts Per Serving:

- Calories: 238 kcal
- Total Fat: 22.2g
- Total Carbs: 2.3g
- Dietary Fiber: 0g
- Net Carbs: 2.3g
- Protein: 5.1g

KALE CHIPS

Serves: 2

Prep time: 10 min

Cook time: 5 min

Ingredients:

- 3 tsp of olive oil
- 12 pieces of kale leaves
- Salt and pepper, as needed

Directions:

1. Preheat oven to 350°F or 175°C.
2. Line a baking sheet with parchment paper.
3. Wash and thoroughly dry kale leaves and place them on the baking sheet.
4. Drizzle kale with olive oil and sprinkle with salt and pepper.
5. Bake 10 to 15 minutes.
6. Serve.

Nutrition Facts Per Serving:

- Calories: 107 kcal
- Total Fat: 7.64g
- Total Carbs: 8.4g
- Dietary Fiber: 3.5g
- Net Carbs: 4.9g
- Protein: 4.11g

KETO BROWNIES

Serves: 16

Prep time: 15 min

Cook time: 10 min

Ingredients:

- 1 cup almond butter
- 3 large eggs
- 170g powdered erythritol
- 100g unsweetened cocoa powder
- ½ tsp baking powder
- ¼ tsp kosher salt

Directions:

1. Preheat oven to 325°F or 165°C.
2. Using a food processor, blend the almond butter and Erythritol for about 2 minutes.
3. Add in the eggs, cocoa powder, baking powder, and a ¼ teaspoon of salt. Blend until smooth.

4. Grease the baking pan.
5. Transfer the batter into the baking pan, and bake for 12 minutes.
6. Let cool for 30 minutes before cutting into desired size.
7. Enjoy!

Nutrition Facts Per Serving:

- Calories: 136 kcal
- Total Fat: 12.54g
- Total Carbs: 4.71g
- Dietary Fiber: 0.5g
- Net Carbs: 4.21g
- Protein: 1.6g

KETO CREAM CHEESE PANCAKE

Serves: 1

Prep time: 5 min

Cook time: 10 min

Ingredients:

- 2 eggs
- 2 ounces cream cheese
- 1 tbsp coconut flour
- ½ tsp cinnamon
- ½ to 1 packet stevia

Directions:

1. Beat or blend together the ingredients until the batter is smooth and free of lumps.
2. Two pancakes is equivalent to one serving. On medium-high, heat up a non-stick skillet or pan with coconut oil or salted butter.
3. Ladle the batter on to the pan. Heat until bubbles

begin to form on top. Flip over, and cook until the other side is sufficiently browned.
4. Serve. Top with sugar-free maple syrup and grass-fed butter.

Nutrition Facts per Serving:

- Calories: 365 kcal
- Total Fat: 29 g
- Total Carbs: 8 g
- Dietary Fiber: 3 g
- Net Carbs: 5 g
- Protein: 17 g

KETO PIZZA CHIPS

Serves: 8

Prep time: 10 min

Cook time: 5 min

Ingredients:

- 10 oz sliced pepperoni
- 1 (8 oz) bag shredded mozzarella cheese
- 1 (8 oz) bag shredded Parmesan cheese
- 2 tsp Italian seasoning

Directions:

1. Preheat oven to 400°F or 200°C.
2. Line two cookie sheets with aluminum foil, and place the pepperoni on the sheets.
3. Sprinkle with shredded mozzarella cheese, grated parmesan, and Italian seasoning.
4. Bake for 8-10 minutes.

5. Remove and let cool for about 5 minutes or until crispy.
6. Serve with marinara if you like.

Nutrition Facts Per Serving:

- Calories: 250 kcal
- Total Fat: 18.9g
- Total Carbs: 2.65g
- Dietary Fiber: 0.3g
- Net Carbs: 2.35g
- Protein: 16.18g

LOW-CARB SOUR CREAM BLUEBERRY MUFFIN

This protein-packed breakfast food item can satisfy you throughout the morning. Serve with a bit of grass-fed butter on top, or enjoy this muffin with bacon or eggs. These muffins are a perfect way to power up your day.

Serves: 15

Prep time: 15 min

Cook time: 20 min

Ingredients:

- 2 cups almond flour
- ½ tsp baking soda
- ¼ cup Erythritol
- 1 cup sour cream
- ½ tsp salt
- 2 eggs
- 4 ounces blueberries, fresh
- 1/8 cup butter, melted

Directions:

Preheat the oven to 350°F (175°C). Place cupcake papers inside the individual muffin holes of your muffin tin.

In a large bowl, whisk together the dry ingredients and the almond flour.

In another bowl, beat the eggs lightly. Add in the butter and sour cream. Mix until thoroughly combined.

Combine the almond flour mixture with the sour cream mixture. Stir until thoroughly mixed. Add the blueberries until they are evenly incorporated.

Spoon the batter into the muffin cups, and fill each muffin paper up to ½ full.

Bake the muffins until golden or for about 20 minutes.

Allow to slightly cool. Serve hot with butter.

Nutrition Facts per Serving:

Total Carbs: 5 g

Dietary Fiber: 2 g

Net Carbs: 3 g

Total Fat: 13 g

Protein: 5 g

Calories: 147 kcal

PARMESAN CHIPS

Serves: 4

Prep time: 10 min

Cook time: 15 min

Ingredients:

- 6 oz grated Parmesan cheese
- 4 tbsp almond flour
- 1 tsp rosemary
- ½ tsp garlic powder

Directions:

1. Start by heating your oven to 350°F or 180°C.
2. Mix Parmesan cheese and almond flour in a medium bowl.
3. Add rosemary and garlic powder, and continue to mix everything together.
4. Place each tablespoon of cheese mixture on a baking sheet.

5. Bake for 10-15 minutes.
6. Let cool before serving.

Nutrition Facts Per Serving:

- Calories: 227 kcal
- Total Fat: 16g
- Total Carbs: 8g
- Dietary Fiber: 1g
- Net Carbs: 7g
- Protein: 13.9g

PEANUT BUTTER COOKIE

Serves: 12

Prep time: 15 min

Cook time: 10 min

Ingredients:

- 1 cup peanut butter
- ½ cup powdered erythritol
- 1 egg

Directions:

1. Preheat oven to 350°F or 175°C.
2. In a medium bowl, combine the peanut butter, erythritol and the egg. Mix well.
3. Form the cookie dough into 1-inch balls.
4. Place the balls on a parchment paper lined baking sheet.
5. Press down on a dough with a fork twice in opposite directions. Repeat with the rest of the doughs.

6. Bake for about 12 minutes.
7. Let cool for 5 minutes before serving.

Nutrition Facts Per Serving:

- Calories: 80 kcal
- Total Fat: 5.12g
- Total Carbs: 7.46g
- Dietary Fiber: 1.5g
- Net Carbs: 5.96g
- Protein: 2.91g

PECAN PEANUT BUTTER BARS

Serves: 12

Prep time: 5 min

Cook time: 60 min

Ingredients:

- 2 cups pecans
- ½ cup coconut oil
- ½ cup peanut butter
- 1 tsp vanilla extract
- 4 small plastic containers or muffin cups

Directions:

1. Measure out your pecans into 4 individual dishes. About ½ cup pecans per dish.
2. Combine peanut butter and coconut oil in a microwave safe bowl.
3. Microwave about 30 seconds. Stir. Repeat until melted.

4. Add vanilla extract to the mixture. Mix well.
5. Pour ¼ cup of the melted mixture over each container with pecans. Make sure all of the nuts are covered by the mixture.
6. Put in the refrigerator until set, about 1 hour.

Nutrition Facts Per Serving:

- Calories: 225 kcal
- Total Fat: 22.91g
- Total Carbs: 5.81g
- Dietary Fiber: 1.8g
- Net Carbs: 4.01
- Protein: 2.31g

LOW-CARB DRINKS AND SMOOTHIES (5 RECIPES)

AVOCADO COCONUT MILK SHAKE

Serves: 1

Prep time: 5 min

Cook time: 0 min

Ingredients:

- ½ avocado
- ½ cups Unsweetened Coconut Milk
- 5 drops stevia
- 5 Ice Cubes

Directions:

1. Add all the ingredients to the blender.
2. Blend until smooth.

Nutrition Facts Per Serving:

- Calories: 437 kcal

- Total Fat: 43.34g
- Total Carbs: 20.2g
- Dietary Fiber: 9.4g
- Net Carbs: 10.8g
- Protein: 4.76g

BULLETPROOF COFFEE

Serves: 1

Prep time: 5 min

Cook time: 10 min

Ingredients:

- 1 cup water
- 2 tbsp coffee
- 1 tbsp grass fed butter
- 1 tbsp coconut oil
- ¼ tsp vanilla extract

Directions:

1. Brew coffee your preferred way.
2. Add butter and coconut oil to the blender.
3. Pour the coffee into the blender.
4. Add the vanilla extract and blend for 20 seconds.

Nutrition Facts Per Serving:

- Calories: 284 kcal
- Total Fat: 24.43g
- Total Carbs: 0.14g
- Dietary Fiber: 0g
- Net Carbs: 0.14g
- Protein: 16.54g

CREAMY AVOCADO CACAO CHIA SHAKE

Serves: 1

Prep time: 15 min

Cook time: 0 min

Ingredients:

- ½ avocado
- 1 tbsp chia seeds
- ½ oz 70% dark chocolate
- 1 cup unsweetened almond milk
- 5 ice cubes

Directions:

1. Mix the chia seeds with the unsweetened almond milk and wait for 10 minutes.
2. Add all the ingredients to the blender.
3. Blend until smooth.
4. Topped with some chopped dark chocolate.

Nutrition Facts Per Serving:

- Calories: 533 kcal
- Total Fat: 37.5g
- Total Carbs: 38.72g
- Dietary Fiber: 18.1g
- Net Carbs: 20.62g
- Protein: 15.5g

FROZEN BERRY SHAKE

Serves: 1

Prep time: 10 min

Cook time: 0 min

Ingredients:

- A handful of ice cubes
- 1 cup unsweetened coconut milk
- 1 tsp vanilla extract
- ½ cup of frozen blueberries
- ½ cup of frozen raspberries
- ½ cup of frozen strawberries

Directions:

1. Combine all the ingredients in a blender.
2. Process for about a minute or two.
3. Serve.

Nutrition Facts Per Serving:

- Calories: 276 kcal
- Total Fat: 9.05g
- Total Carbs: 40.07g
- Dietary Fiber: 9g
- Net Carbs: 27.53g
- Protein: 9.33g

PEANUT BUTTER SHAKE

Serves: 1

Prep time: 10 min

Cook time: 0 min

Ingredients:

- 1 cup unsweetened almond milk
- 2 tbsp peanut butter
- 1 scoop chocolate protein powder
- 4 drops vanilla extract
- 2 tbsp heavy cream
- 5 ice cubes

Directions:

1. Add all the ingredients to the blender.
2. Blend until smooth.

Nutrition Facts Per Serving:

- Calories: 519 kcal
- Total Fat: 27.35g
- Total Carbs: 33.43g
- Dietary Fiber: 3.7g
- Net Carbs: 29.3g
- Protein: 35.5g

BONUS FAT BOMBS RECIPES (6 RECIPES)

COCONUT KETO CANDY

If you love candy and coconut, then you're sure to love this coconut-rich candy. Remember that an ice cube tray will work in a pinch, but you can make it more decorative with silicone molds of your choice. Add a little more sugar substitute if you want it to be a little sweeter. Just remember that you'll need to melt your coconut oil in advance, and virgin coconut oil would be the healthiest choice.

Serves: 10

Prep Time: 5 min

Total Time: 15 min

Ingredients:

- ⅓ Cup Coconut Butter, Softened
- ⅓ Cup Coconut Oil, Melted
- 1 Ounce Shredded Coconut, Unsweetened
- 1 Teaspoon Sugar Substitute

Directions:

1. Start by mixing all of your ingredients together, and make sure that the sugar substitute is well dissolved.
2. Pour into silicone molds, and then refrigerate for about an hour.

Nutrition Facts per Serving:

- Calories: 104 kcal
- Total Fat: 11 g
- Total Carbs: 0.8 g
- Dietary Fiber: 0.2 g
- Net Carbs: 0.6 g
- Protein: 0.3 g

CRUNCHY AVOCADO BOMBS

Avocados are full of healthy fats, which work perfectly for this recipe. You'll find that with a dash of pecan, it has just enough flavor to make it mouthwatering.

The best part of this recipe is that with three ingredients, it's incredibly simple, and it has a texture that you're sure to love.

Serves: 8

Prep Time: 5 min

Total Time: 15 min

Ingredients:

- 6 Pecans
- 2 Avocados
- 4 Slices Bacon

Directions:

1. Cook your bacon in a pan over medium-high heat until the bacon is crispy.

2. Take it off of heat, allowing it to cool before crumbling it.
3. Take a bowl and mash your avocados, and then crumble your pecans.
4. Mix all ingredients together, and make round balls using an ice cream scooper.

Nutrition Facts per Serving:

- Calories: 151 kcal
- Total Fat: 14.27 g
- Total Carbs: 4.74 g
- Dietary Fiber: 3.6 g
- Net Carbs: 1.14 g
- Protein: 2.86 g

KETO PARMESAN PESTO DIP

This dip is great to serve with crisp lettuce or cucumber sticks. You can also try it with kale if you want a crisp, bitter crunch. It tastes better cold, but it can be served at room temperature as well.

Serves: 6 (about two tablespoons)

Prep Time: 5 min

Total Time: 5 min

Ingredients:

- 1 Cup Full Fat Cream Cheese
- 2 Tablespoons Basil Pesto
- ½ Cup Parmesan Cheese, Grated
- 8 Olives, Sliced
- Salt and Pepper to Taste

Directions:

1. Mix all of your ingredients together in a mixing bowl.

2. Refrigerate for at least 20 minutes before serving.

<u>Nutrition Facts per Serving:</u>

- Calories: 161 kcal
- Total Fat: 14.33 g
- Total Carbs: 3.43 g
- Dietary Fiber: 0.2 g
- Net Carbs: 3.23 g
- Protein: 5.42 g

MINTY CHOCOLATE FAT BOMBS

These are multi-layered fat bombs with one amazing layer of pure mint and other layers of a chocolate minty goodness that will melt in your mouth. You can make your own chocolate with cocoa powder and coconut oil, whipping it together. Though, if you have 85% dark chocolate, then that is allowed as well.

Serves: 6

Prep Time: 10 min

Total Time: 20 min

Ingredients:

- ½ Cup Coconut Oil, Melted
- 2 Tablespoons Cocoa Powder
- 1 Tablespoon Granulated Stevia (or sweetener of choice)
- ½ Teaspoon Peppermint Essence

Directions:

1. Start by melting your coconut oil, and adding your peppermint essence and sweetener.
2. Add cocoa powder to half of the mixture and mix well in another bowl.
3. Pour the chocolate mixture into the silicone molds, and then place them in the fridge. Refrigerate for 5-10 minutes.
4. Make the mint layer by pouring the mint mixture into the silicon molds. Refrigerate for another 5-10 minutes.
5. Pour the last layer of chocolate mixture into the molds. Refrigerate and let harden.

Nutrition Facts per Serving:

- Calories: 161 kcal
- Total Fat: 18.5 g
- Total Carbs: 1.15 g
- Dietary Fiber: 0.7 g
- Net Carbs: 0.45 g
- Protein: 0.4 g

SOUR CREAM BACON DIP

With both cream cheese and sour cream, this dip is smooth and rich in flavor. It's a perfect fat bomb as well as a party dip.

Serves: 12

Prep Time: 5-10 min

Total Time: 40 min

Ingredients:

- 5 Slices Bacon, Cooked & Crumbled
- 1½ Cups Sour Cream
- 1 Cup Cream Cheese
- 1 Cup Cheddar Cheese, Shredded
- 1 Cup Scallions, Sliced

Directions:

1. Start by heating your oven to 400 degrees F (200 degrees C).

2. Combine all of your ingredients together in a bowl, and then spoon out onto a baking dish.
3. Cook for 25 to 35 minutes. The cheese should be bubbling when it's done.
4. Let it cool slightly before serving.

Nutrition Facts per Serving:

- Calories: 190 kcal
- Total Fat: 16.76 g
- Total Carbs: 3.5 g
- Dietary Fiber: 0.2 g
- Net Carbs: 3.3 g
- Protein: 6.58 g

STRAWBERRY CHEESECAKE MINIS

Cream cheese is your best friend when it comes to fat bombs, and these strawberry cheesecake minis are no different. They'll make sure that you aren't missing strawberry cheesecake just for choosing a healthier diet. If you want a slightly richer flavor, then add a little more vanilla. Also, if you don't have fresh strawberries on hand, frozen strawberries will work, too. I prefer to keep them frozen, but storing them in your refrigerator will work as well.

Serves: 8

Prep Time: 5 min

Total Time: 15-20 min

Ingredients:

- ½ Cup Strawberries, Fresh & Mashed
- ¾ Cup Cream Cheese, Softened
- ¼ Cup Coconut Oil, Softened
- 10-15 Drops Liquid Stevia
- 1 Teaspoon Vanilla Extract

Directions:

1. Start by combining all of the ingredients in a bowl, and mixing with a hand mixer until completely smooth. You can also do this in a high-speed blender.
2. Spoon into mini muffin tins, and place in the freezer. It'll take about two hours to set, and then you can place them in the fridge.

Nutritional Facts per Serving:

- Calories: 129 kcal
- Total Fat: 13.27 g
- Total Carbs: 1.55 g
- Dietary Fiber: 0.2 g
- Net Carbs: 1.35 g
- Protein: 1.66 g

FAT BOMBS - MORE RECIPES

IF YOU'RE INTERESTED IN GETTING MORE FAT BOMBS recipes, I have written a **Fat Bombs Cookbook** with **over 30 most amazing fat bombs**. Don't hesitate to look for Fat bombs by Andrea J. Clark on Amazon!

AFTERWORD

Now that you're armed with all the information, you've read the tips and tricks, and you know the secret of Intermittent Fasting Keto, are you ready to make the commitment?

Imagine yourself in 6 months. What do you see? Do you see the same old you, overweight and unhappy? Sick and tired? Or do you want to see a more energetic and happier version of yourself? This is within your grasp, all you have to do is let go of your old way of thinking and embrace Intermittent Fasting Keto.

With the Intermittent Fasting Keto diet, you can reclaim control of your body and your life. You can learn to love food again, all while losing weight and building a faster metabolism. You can have the body and the life you dream of if you're willing to work for it.

The journey won't be easy. It will have its ups and downs, but if you can commit to the new lifestyle, I know you will be able to reach your goals.

I truly hope that this book has been able to help you to

make the transition easier. Commit to the new lifestyle and watch yourself transform to a better, more confident person.

Good luck!

Andrea

AUTHOR'S NOTE

Thank you so much for taking the time to read my book. I hope you have enjoyed reading this book as much as I've enjoyed writing it. If you enjoyed this book, please consider leaving a review on Amazon. Your support really means a lot and keeps me going.

If you have any questions, please don't hesitate to contact me at ask@cleaneatingspirit.com

Follow me on Facebook or Instagram for more information:

Facebook: https://www.facebook.com/cleaneatingspirit

Instagram: https://www.instagram.com/cleaneatingspirit

Made in the USA
San Bernardino, CA
14 July 2018